For Ariela, always my bright light.

TELLING SILENCES
A DOCTOR'S TALES OF DENIAL

HILLEL HALKIN MD

Copyright © 2013 Hillel Halkin MD
All rights reserved.
ISBN: 1490423524
ISBN 13: 9781490423524

This book is dedicated to my patients, my colleagues and my students from whom I have learnt so much.

The identities of patients and their families have been thoroughly altered so as to render them unrecognizable.

TABLE OF CONTENTS

INTRODUCTION vii

1. GUILT(Y) OR NOT 1

2. DOUBLE CROSSED 21

3. MEDICAL MEDLEY 41

4. MULTIPLE VEILS 67

5. HEROES DON'T CRY 85

6. IN TANDEM 107

7. PENANCE 123

8. SHUTTERED LISTENERS 141

9. MY OWN MEDICINE 167

INTRODUCTION

At the approach of danger there are always two voices that speak with equal force in the heart of man: one very reasonably tells the man to consider the nature of the danger and the means of avoiding it; the other even more reasonable says that it is too painful and harassing to think of the danger, since it is not a man's power to provide for everything and escape from the general march of events; and that it is therefore better to turn aside from the painful subject till it has come, and to think of what is pleasant.

—Leo Tolstoy, *War and Peace*

For decades, if not centuries, doctors have been taught the crucial importance of communication with patients in ensuring an optimal outcome to the medical encounter. More recently, patients are increasingly encouraged to be directly involved in the decisions about or choice of their own treatment options; their family members too are often active participants in this process. These developments presuppose an open and unimpeded flow of frank, full, and accurate information among all players. However, in more than fifty years in medicine, I have come to realize that assumed good communication is not always what it seems. Barriers, discernible or hidden, conscious or unconscious, often stand in the way, rendering communication at best incomplete, or at worst actually misleading.

My aim in writing this book is to impart recognition of these barriers and their potentially dire consequences. *Telling Silences* comprises a selection of strange clinical tales that continue to haunt me after all these years. They are all true stories of patients, their family members, or their physicians, as well as of physicians as patients. Their common thread is that they all depict how processes of denial or altered cognition, engendered by the painful realities or threatening implications of illness, created unrecognized barriers that disrupted communication between doctor and patient, seriously impeding proper transfer of relevant information so vital to the successful rendering of a diagnosis or treatment decision.

Some of these stories portray other aspects of these barriers. They depict physicians as biased caregivers, choosing to ignore details related by the patient or opinions voiced by colleagues that did not fit in with their preconceived ideas. In other cases, I found that physicians, upon becoming patients themselves, were just as prone to deny their own conditions, as were their patients or family members.

While all these tales begin with a patient's complaint, silences in the telling veil a vast, unknown world from the doctor, rendering the road to diagnosis and cure or management circuitous or leading to a dead end. Treatment may be off the mark in ways that range from the merely ineffective to the downright disastrous.

Making these silences speak in retrospect may perhaps sharpen my humbling recognition of flaws in my own listening and highlight the limitations of our professional hearing aids. Modern medicine has become overwhelmingly technological. Patients take their various body systems to specialists whose practices are procedure driven. Generalists

INTRODUCTION

too spend most of their limited interview time facing their computer screens rather than looking at the patient as they try to listen to what is being said and at the same time complete the required electronic record. Sadly, they can no longer be expected to seek nuanced clues in the patient's narrative, to listen, so to speak, with their "third ear," the term coined by the Freudian psychoanalyst Theodor Reik nearly sixty-five years ago. It is my hope that somehow coming generations of physicians will—at least—retain or rediscover the importance of the two ears they already have.

1.

GUILT(Y) OR NOT

The writing of this memoir—and its principal subject matter—owes much to a powerful recollection of mine going back some twenty years. In 1993 I was asked by a well-known Tel Aviv law firm to serve as an expert witness in a court case concerning a forty-six-year-old man who had died suddenly of a heart attack three months earlier. His widow was planning to sue the general practitioner and the HMO the doctor worked for (the largest in the country) for what she believed had been negligent mismanagement of her late husband's illness, and the attorneys wanted me to meet her and review the facts. Naturally, all the medical records they were now retrieving would be put at my disposal as soon as they were in hand.

A few days later, I met Anna at my office. She was a good-looking, well-dressed, and vivacious woman, probably in her early forties. Her wide-set, dark eyes seemed to look out on the world inquisitively, although at that moment I detected mainly sadness and anger in them.

I invited her to make herself comfortable in the sitting area of my office.

"I was sorry to hear of your loss," I began. "How are you coping, and in what way do you think I can help you?"

"I suppose I'm all right," she said, slowly considering my question. "With everything that's happened, I suppose you could say that. My sons are back at school, and I'm working again."

"What kind of work do you do?" I asked.

"I handcraft costume jewelry in my basement workshop at home. My stuff has always been quite popular. People come to the house to see the new creations. They're actually buying more now than before," she added wryly. "They probably think I need the money more now than before Sam died. I suppose that's not entirely wrong; raising my two boys, twelve and sixteen years old, on my own is not going to be easy."

Picking up on that note, I said, "I hope you don't mind my asking, but how are you set up financially, now that you're alone?"

"Please understand," she quickly replied, "it's not money that brings me here. Sam was an insurance agent. His life insurance policies left us well cared for. If only he'd looked after himself as well as he did us," she added bitterly.

"Then why are you here?" I asked. "Why do you need the hassle of this lawsuit you're contemplating? I'm sure you know how difficult and unpleasant it's going to be. It can get very nasty for you and really difficult for your sons."

At that Anna rose to her feet and stood squarely in front of where I was sitting, her face suffused with emotion.

"I'm here because they killed Sam!" she exclaimed. "I want them to pay for their negligence. I also want to save other miserable souls from suffering the same fate at their hands. Nothing will deter me from going through with this case."

It appeared that her determination was unshakable, and I realized that she really was out to crucify the doctors who had treated her husband. It was clearly not a matter of money, as were so many of these malpractice suits. I decided to determine the facts as she saw them.

"I understand. Please tell me a little about your husband. Any detail you could tell me about his illness and treatment would help me better understand why you have reached the conclusion that it was so grossly mishandled. Please don't leave anything out, even if it should seem unimportant or irrelevant. Sometimes it is the small things that give one insight into the larger picture."

She thought for a moment and then began to recall.

"Sam was a serious type, not given to too many words, but with a fine sense of humor. He was a hard worker, kept long hours, with little free time for me or our sons. He was not particularly interested in his appearance—or his health, for that matter, as things turned out. He ate too much, was overweight, and did little in the way of exercising. He was diagnosed with mild diabetes in 1987 by a private specialist who put him on pills that I don't think he took regularly, despite my hassling him. He was proud of his nonchalance and even jokingly boasted of never going for routine checkups and of having seen his HMO GP only once, during a severe bout of flu, years ago. I suspect that he even went on smoking cigarettes at work after I had put my foot down and made him quit—at least at home, where I had some control. There, I was the homemaker and everyone's organizer. I was never at a loss for time for the boys and for Sam, in particular, whenever there was a little interlude for us."

This was said with some pride as she looked at me, obviously expecting approval. I nodded and asked her to continue.

"I've always been a bit of a health freak, and Sam's lifestyle and habits were a constant source of concern to me. I knew that his lack of exercise, overeating, and excess weight were bad. The cigarettes were even worse, seeing that his father too had been diabetic and had had heart disease for years. 'Why don't you get a medical checkup?' I had often pleaded with him. 'I don't need one,' he used to say. 'All my friends spend their time going to doctors, getting checkups for their various symptoms. I don't see that it does them much good. It just gets them constantly worried, not to mention the pressure it puts on their wives and children. Every checkup generates more checkups. I firmly believe that once those doctors start looking for something, they sure as hell will find it. So I would much rather not get on that carousel because I might not be able to get off.' He smiled as he said this and ruffled my hair, telling me to stop fretting. 'Don't worry, I am going to stay healthy and be around for many years so that you can go on nagging me.'"

Anna paused and looked at me as if asking for a reaction. I just nodded once more, waiting for the rest of the story.

"I actually felt that he was proud of never going to see a doctor. As you must have guessed by now, I'm not one who gives up very easily. I harassed him incessantly to quit smoking. I made calorie-counting a rule for all our meals at home, hoping to get him to lose his excess weight. Most of all, I tried to get Sam into an exercising mode. As I told you, I've always been really keen on physical exercise. I went to the gym regularly and jogged at least an hour a day. Don't ask me how we managed to live together with such conflicting attitudes toward lifestyle and health issues. Anyway, my haranguing was finally partially successful. I got him to join me in walking our Alsatian in the early mornings, at least three times a week." Anna had tears in her eyes as she recounted her efforts to save Sam from himself.

"Did he keep up the walks?" I asked.

"Yes, he did. Despite his initial protests and moans and groans, it seemed, after a few weeks, that he was actually beginning to enjoy the outings. The aftereffects of the physical effort were exhilarating, and he was pleased with the slight dip in his weight for the first time in years. He even conceded that he ought to start thinking about doing something about his away-from-home smoking habit and promised to lose more weight by being more careful about what he ate at the office."

"What about the checkup you wanted him to have?" I asked.

"He always joked about all those losers sitting outside doctors' offices at the HMO clinics. 'Is that where you want to see me, sitting in line?' he would ask."

"It seems that you really started a professional preventive health program for him," I commented.

"Yes, I certainly did. I gradually increased the pace of our walking. After a month or so, we were covering a three-kilometer distance in about forty-five minutes, not a bad pace at all. But that was when the trouble started." Anna stopped abruptly.

"What trouble?" I asked.

Anna hesitated, unable to resume the flow of words. I offered her a glass of water, which she gulped down. She then continued.

"By now it was early December. The mornings were getting quite cold, and Sam first noticed some discomfort in his chest after thirty minutes or so of our brisk walking. He thought it was the cold. The sensation of discomfort subsided when he slowed down for a minute or two and did not reappear, even when he accelerated his step again. At first, Sam put it down to his being in such poor physical shape, coupled with the cold air he wasn't used to. I could shoot myself today, because neither he nor I thought it was a signal of things to come."

Anna paused and took a deep breath, almost a sigh.

"Please go on," I said.

"The discomfort waxed and waned for about two weeks, but then things got worse. It was taking less time and a far slower pace to produce the pain. It was also taking longer for it to subside, and it now tended to recur when we continued the walk. One morning the pressure in Sam's chest started only minutes after we took off, making him stop, then, after a motionless few minutes, slowly turn around and return home. Following him, it was only then that I realized something serious was going on. I put my foot down.

"'You are coming with me right now to see Dr. Rosen, 'I said. 'I can't go now, I have a meeting in town, but I will go this afternoon,' he promised. 'You give me your word?' I insisted. Sam got angry. 'I said I would go, and I will. Now let me get changed. I have to go to work, and I can't cope with your nagging me this morning.'"

Anna recalled that he left the house in a temper.

"And did he go to see the doctor?" I asked.

"Yes, he did. I made sure by phoning the HMO clinic to make an appointment for that afternoon and then phoned Sam to tell him it was set for four o'clock. I couldn't be there because I had to take my younger son to his swimming training session, but Sam promised me that he would report the entire story faithfully to the doctor. As I mentioned, he'd been to see this doctor only once before, three years earlier, during a bad bout of flu, and the doctor didn't really know him. So I was a bit worried that Sam would gloss over his condition and persuade the doctor that there was nothing really wrong."

Anna paused, straining to remember every detail of that afternoon.

"And what did Sam tell you when he came home that evening?" I asked.

"He told me that Dr. Rosen had been called away that afternoon and that he had been seen by another doctor, Dr. Abrahams. After hearing the details of Sam's story, Dr. Abrahams told him that he suspected the pain may have been related to a heart problem, possibly angina pectoris," Anna related.

Not an unlikely assumption, I thought, given the story related by such a heavy man, and a smoker to boot.

"Did the doctor prescribe any medication for Sam?" I asked Anna.

"No. Dr. Abrahams wanted to be sure of his diagnosis first, so he had not prescribed any medication yet. He had scheduled a consultation for Sam with a cardiologist and an exercise stress test for two days later. Meanwhile, he had advised Sam to cut down his smoking load and slow the pace of the morning walks," Anna remembered.

"How did Sam react to this advice?" I asked.

"Well, he wasn't very happy about Dr. Abrahams's recommendation for him to see a dietician as soon as possible. It appears that the doctor had voiced concern over Sam's twenty-kilogram excess weight. Sam never liked to discuss his weight. He loved eating, you see." Anna's voice broke for a moment.

In view of Sam's apparent reticence in discussions of his health, I asked Anna whether, in her opinion, Sam had truthfully reported to the doctor the latest developments during his morning walks with her.

"I asked him point-blank if he had described the worsening of his symptoms over the last few days," she answered. "Sam had responded, again somewhat angrily, 'Well, of course I did, most definitely. Why would I go to the doctor in the first place if not to consult him about my symptoms? What would be the point in wasting his time and mine? You don't think I'd play around with such serious problems, do you? I even told him that I had not been able to even begin our usual walk early this morning.'"

"Did you believe Sam?" I asked.

"Yes, I did. He was very definite," she said with conviction.

"Did Dr. Abrahams examine Sam with his stethoscope?"

"No. I asked Sam about that," she said.

"Did he do an electrocardiogram?"

"No. Sam said the doctor had told him that further examination would be done thoroughly by the cardiologist to whom he was referring him. He assured Sam that he need not worry, that the situation was not that urgent, and that he was lucky to have gotten a consultation slot so quickly since the waiting lists are usually eight to ten days long."

Anna told me that she had not been reassured by all this and had continued probing. She had asked Sam again if the doctor had been worried about their walks, whether he had told the doctor that the pain was getting worse these last few days, and if he'd mentioned that it was taking far less of an effort to produce the pain now, that it now took much longer for the pain to subside than when they had first noticed it several weeks earlier.

Sam had assured her that he had given the doctor all the relevant information in great detail. Actually, the doctor had praised him for having started an exercise program and wanted him to continue, though at a pace slower than that which caused the pressure on his chest. The doctor was not prescribing any medication yet, Sam had told Anna, because he wanted to avoid any drugs that could affect the ECG tracings during the stress test, possibly masking signs of coronary artery disease, the cause of angina pectoris and heart attacks. They would discuss treatment right after getting the cardiologist's opinion and recommendations.

At this point, Anna recounted, Sam had become angry and impatient with her.

"'I want you to stop this interrogation,' he said. 'You've already made me miss two afternoon meetings. I did what you wanted and went to see the doctor. I'm sure he knows what he's doing, so please stop worrying so much. I can't stand all this harassing. Let's talk about this tomorrow, if you wish.' At that point he switched on the TV and refused to talk any further."

"What happened then?" I asked, knowing that the most painful part of the story was about to unfold.

Anna took a deep breath and began to relate the events of that night.

"We went to sleep fairly early. Around midnight Sam woke up with a very strong pain in his chest and within minutes was short of breath and covered in cold sweat. I realized immediately the seriousness of his condition and phoned for the emergency ambulance. The ambulance team arrived within ten minutes. It took them no longer than another ten minutes to start an IV drip, hook him up to an ECG monitor, and get him into the ambulance. By this time Sam was only semiconscious.

"On the way to the hospital, with sirens howling outside, the paramedic told me that the outlook was grave. Sam was in the throes of a heart attack, quite massive too, he said. He was in radiophone contact with the ER cardiologist, and they were administering a blood-thinning drug to try to dissolve the clot that was probably blocking one of the arteries supplying blood to the heart muscle. But the blood pressure was very low and not rising, despite the other medications going into his vein. At the hospital, fifteen minutes later, as Sam was wheeled rapidly into the ICU, the cardiology resident rushing in with him could only say, 'He's in a bad way, Mrs. T., he's in shock. I hope we can pull him out of it.'"

Anna fell silent. I could imagine the shock that she was reliving now in the telling. Many family members of patients have described to me the moment of realization that their loved one was not going to pull through as a sensation of the familiar world suddenly caving in around them, and a sense of unreality encroaching on the everyday world moving around them in its usual ceaseless, uncaring motion.

"Please go on. I know it is difficult for you, but every detail is important to your case," I gently prodded.

"I was in the waiting room, watching nurses rush in and out, bringing equipment and taking it away again. No one would tell me what was happening. Finally, an hour later, the cardiologist reappeared. Looking at his face, I knew immediately what he was about to say—'I'm truly sorry, Mrs. T., we did everything we could. It was a massive coronary. The damage to the heart muscle was so extensive, he was in shock and then in cardiac arrest. It was just too late; we couldn't bring him back.'"

That was Anna's story. The questions she then asked me were right to the point.

"Given my husband's symptoms, shouldn't the HMO doctor have recognized the imminent gravity of the situation? Shouldn't he have at least listened to his heart with his stethoscope? Shouldn't he have done an ECG recording there and then? Shouldn't he have referred him to hospital immediately? Barring that, shouldn't he at least have prescribed appropriate medications immediately, possibly averting the heart attack that occurred only hours later, or reducing its severity? Couldn't his death have been prevented?"

She was probably right, I thought to myself.

"I completely understand your thoughts and questions, and I am deeply sorry for what you've been through. Let me get the medical records the lawyers have requisitioned. We'll probably talk again before I can say whether I can help you or not," I said, accompanying her to the door.

I knew, however, even then, that I was going to take on the case. It seemed open and shut, requiring no sophisticated or highly specialized medical knowledge.

There are two types of effort-induced chest pain related to the heart, known as angina pectoris. Both are caused by obstructions to blood flow through the coronary arteries, which feed the heart muscle with the oxygen it needs. The first, stable angina pectoris, is characterized by a pretty regular pattern of chest pain over time. It is brought on by the same degree of physical effort, manifests with the same severity, and disappears in the same number of minutes when the effort is stopped. It never occurs at rest. This type can be dealt with without excess haste, in terms of diagnostic procedures and treatment, as it is usually not a harbinger of an imminent heart attack.

The second type, unstable angina, is characterized by a recent onset and a pattern of increasing severity. Less and less effort brings on the pain, more time is required for the pain to subside, and the pain may occur even at rest. Unstable angina is a medical emergency, as it indicates a very high likelihood of an impending heart attack. It requires immediate and aggressive hospital treatment, using appropriate drugs, very early coronary angiography, and consideration of invasive treatment of the coronary blockage, either by means of balloon dilatation and stenting or by directly proceeding to coronary bypass surgery.

All this is canonical, drummed into the mind of any well-trained medical student, intern, or resident physician in training. The key to the correct diagnosis, even if still only suspected, is to elicit the information needed for the distinction between the two types of angina pectoris. This is done by simply asking the appropriate questions while taking the medical history of any patient complaining of effort-related chest pain. It seemed inconceivable to me that given the story, as recounted by Anna, the physician could have failed to recognize that he was dealing with classic unstable angina. Clearly, this had been the gross error that led to the wrong course of action and contributed to the terrible outcome: Sam's death.

How could the doctor have missed it?

That being said, I knew I had to wait to see the physician's notes in Sam's HMO medical chart, which would surely clarify matters. In the meantime, I got to work on the outline of my expert opinion, enumerating everything that seemed to have gone wrong in the doctor's office that fateful afternoon. The main point, of course, was the physician's failure to recognize the severity of Sam's history, misclassifying it as stable angina. Among the secondary points was his failure to simply do a physical examination. The stethoscope could have indicated blockage of one of the heart valves, which may have served to heighten his suspicion of the severity of Sam's condition. Another was his failing to record an ECG, the machine being standard equipment in all HMO clinics. A normal tracing would not have ruled out unstable angina, but if abnormalities had been found, they would surely have served as a real warning.

Copies of Sam's medical record arrived about a week later. There were only three pages of text: The first, just the front piece with Sam's personal details, address, etc. The second, a brief handwritten note dated 1987, describing a flu-like illness of several days duration, with no follow-up. The third was a preformatted patient interview and physical exam record. The doctor could check itemized boxes or leave them unmarked. Lined space was also provided next to each boxed item for any free text needed. It was immediately obvious that there wasn't much information listed, certainly not as detailed as I had hoped for. Sam's age and body weight were there. His main complaint was a cryptic "chest pain, on walking, started six weeks ago" with no further elaboration. The significant past medical history recorded his smoking habit and his years of being overweight. The physical exam portion of the form showed the blood pressure as 145/90. The box for examination of the heart was checked as "no significant findings," and no other details were listed. The physician's assessment was brief: "Effort-related chest pain, possible angina pectoris, two months' duration, risk factors: obesity, smoking, possible hypertension." The plan for further management: "Exercise stress test and cardiology consult scheduled for December 12. Follow up here December 13."

And that was it. Hardly meticulous or accurate medical record keeping, I thought to myself. At the time, scrupulous note taking wasn't of top priority for the harassed HMO general practitioner with a line of patients queuing for his attention, each able to enjoy only a few minutes of his time when finally admitted to his office. Physicians were not yet aware then of the importance of accurate and complete medical records, not only for the patients' welfare, but also for their own protection, in case of future lawsuits. However, as I wasn't being asked to evaluate the physician's record-keeping capabilities, I proceeded to write my opinion of what had happened to Sam and why.

It seemed pretty straightforward to me. The history recounted by Sam could not be interpreted by any competent physician as stable angina pectoris. The crescendo nature of the symptoms should have alerted Sam's physician to the more severe alternative, that of unstable angina, with its far more severe potential consequences. This was the major error that had led to the physician's inappropriate course of action—with its dire consequences. Add to that the absence of a physical examination of the heart, the delay in obtaining a simple ECG tracing, the refraining from immediately prescribing simple medication such as aspirin, and it all really couldn't amount to anything other than gross negligence. It wasn't difficult to buttress these thoughts with textbook-level quotations and to put in all in writing, a four-page document I duly sent off to the attorney.

Several months later I heard from the lawyers again. The defense had finally submitted its response to Anna's claim. They were denying any error or mismanagement on the part of Sam's physician. The documents included a deposition given by the physician, answering questions raised by Anna's lawyers. The major argument was that given the information supplied by Sam—or rather the lack of information, as recounted by the physician—the doctor's interpretation and course of action had been appropriate and reasonable.

In the deposition, the physician described a talk with Anna that took place during his condolence visit to the family, on the day after the funeral. She had been reserved, he said, but had spoken to him without animosity or revealing her late husband's dislike of anything to do with doctors, checkups, or hospitals. She was distraught over not having been there, at his office, with Sam. Perhaps, she'd added, things might have turned out differently, knowing Sam's reticence to speak to anyone, let alone a new doctor, a total stranger, about what he considered to be his faults.

The deposition went on to stipulate that the medical notes, though very brief, did in fact reflect accurately the information supplied by Sam, which was minimal at best. The physician stated that he had done a brief physical exam, including taking Sam's blood pressure and listening to his heart, hearing nothing abnormal. In view of the facts at his disposal, he concluded, his assessment of the situation had been correct, and the plan for expedited specialist referral for diagnostic and therapeutic recommendations had been appropriate.

In support of this deposition, the lawyers defending the claim submitted an expert medical opinion, written by a well-known internist, in rebuttal of my own. There was no way, he said, that the doctor could have suspected that he was dealing with unstable angina based on the story told by Sam. Everything known about Sam's attitude toward his medical problems is consistent with his having misled the doctor, albeit unwittingly. In effect, the expert continued, Sam's behavior was a classic example of denial, so commonly manifested by patients or their family members as they try to come to terms with the possibility or reality of serious illness.

Quoting extensively from the medical literature, the expert went on to describe what in medical parlance has become known as the "difficult patient," one who actively interferes with the physician's attempts to establish a normal therapeutic relationship. This pattern is seen in patients who don't cooperate with the doctor, either because they can't or because they don't want to. Some refuse outright to undergo various diagnostic tests recommended, while others may appear to be cooperating but in effect are not. A significant number of patients provide inaccurate or incomplete information to routine questions.

The expert's account continued with a survey of publications on mechanisms underlying the denial phenomenon. According to the prevailing "reactance" theory, illness or imminent incapacitation constitute a perceived threat to an individual's freedom. This generates a motivational state aimed at recapturing the affected freedom and preventing the loss of others. In a medical context, patients' perceptions of threats to their freedom or control may induce total denial of the realities of the situation, as well as noncompliance, under varied pretexts, with a physician's recommendations. Other patients make reasoned decisions about treatments based on their own beliefs, personal circumstances, and the information available to them.

Another major theme that emerged in the expert's discussion of denial involved the interactions among autonomy, self-esteem, and the degree of illness or health as perceived by the patient. Self-esteem is directly correlated with the willingness to seek care, especially as illness increases and autonomy decreases. The individual's perception of health status—as well as the perceived roles of the physician, the patient, and their relationship—motivates the patient to seek, or avoid seeking, health care.

Faced with a severe diagnosis, the analysis continued, many people react initially with a kind of numbed disbelief, which very often assumes the form of denial. In the majority of patients, this reaction is subsequently replaced by other coping responses. Some individuals, however, continue to use denial. While alleviating their psychological distress, they subsequently face the adverse effects of delaying or not complying with recommended treatment.

The expert next focused on the tragic effects of severe illness on a patient's life. It causes a dramatic change in the patient's independence and self-esteem. Patients have to go through different stages of mourning in coming to terms with illness and incapacitation. The first stage is rejection of the situation. Repression and disbelief protect the patient from emotional overstrain. Confrontation is the next step, emotionally as well as mentally. "How could it happen?" "What will my future be like?" "How will I cope?" "Why did it happen to me?" The last stage of coping is acceptance and dealing with the new situation, building up new self-confidence.

Much in the proposed mechanisms of denial, the account concluded, fit in very well with the descriptions of Sam's past neglect of his various medical problems, as described by his widow. He had apparently still been caught up in the first stage of the process. This was why he had inaccurately described his symptoms, misleading the physician into the incorrect diagnostic conclusion and the tragic outcome.

My first reaction to this learned expertise was scornful dismissal. In our age of malpractice litigation of epidemic proportions, physicians are regularly asked by lawyers to render expert opinions in lawsuits filed by patients claiming financial compensation from hospitals, HMOs, and individual physicians and their insurers for injuries ostensibly caused by negligent medical treatment. As large sums of money are involved, remuneration is often a key motivating element for some medical experts recruited by both sides of the dispute. Despite the huge amount of attention devoted to this issue by our professional organizations and societies, and the guidelines they have issued on the ethics of professional testimony in the courtroom, medical expert opinions are still frequently colored to suit the needs of those commissioning them. Here again, I thought, was a colleague actually blaming the patient for his own demise, stating denial as the cause of death.

Yet as I read and reread the new documents and compared them with my own written report, I began to wonder. It had all seemed so straightforward to me at the time, but I did remember, very well indeed, how inexplicable I had found the physician's misinterpretation of Sam's symptoms. It had just never occurred to me that he might have heard a wholly different story than that recounted to me by Anna. But then she had been so emphatic, repeatedly insisting that Sam told her he had given the doctor all the relevant details. I now saw that perhaps she had not been an unbiased reporter. By her own description, she was an organizer, a manager, constantly alert to her husband's tendency to conceal his symptoms. It was so out of character for her to let her husband see the doctor alone. Could it have been Anna's sense of guilt that had generated the passionate anger and frustration she had expressed the first time we met? "I'm here because they killed Sam!" she'd told me. "I want them to pay for their negligence."

It would seem that it all came down to what was really said at the doctor's office that fateful afternoon, known only to the doctor being charged with negligence and the deceased. There were no witnesses. If it came to court, the judge would have to be the one to decide which story to believe. Medical experts would have no say in the matter, beyond what was recorded in the patient's chart. I myself was shaken, no longer knowing what to believe. The truth is never quite so simple or so clear-cut.

I put myself in Dr. Abrahams's place and tried to imagine the scene. Here was this overweight man with a serious complaint that required a course of action, the urgency of which I was to decide. Putting aside the question of the physical exam with a stethoscope, which clearly should have been done, would I have been able to detect something that Dr. Abrahams had missed? Presume that Dr. Abrahams was telling the truth. That Sam had, at best, not been accurate in describing the severity of his symptoms, or even worse, had omitted important details. Would I too have come to the same conclusion, that his angina pectoris was of the stable category and that there was no immediate danger?

This whole book is about listening to the silences and deciphering what the patient is not telling us. Medical practice has changed ever so much since my early days. Technology and computers, along with demands for more "efficient" dealing with increased patient loads, have shortened the time doctors can spend listening to their patients, even looking at them, having to move their gaze from the computer screen and keyboard.

In today's world the HMO doctor has no time to truly listen with a third ear, as Theodor Reik would have us listen to our patients. Listening with Reik's third ear involves tuning in to our own unconscious intuitions about what the patient might be hiding. With a line of patients waiting their turn impatiently outside the doctor's office, there is obviously no chance of providing this kind of attention, so doctors tend to rely more and more on machines to tell them what they need to know about their patients. In Sam's case I will never know whether he did indeed deny the severity of his illness and mislead his doctor or whether the doctor was negligent and used denial as defense, nor will I ever know whether the tragedy could have been avoided. In time I learned from the law firm that the case had not gone to trial and there had been a modest out-of-court settlement.

Decades later I realized what a lingering effect Sam and Anna's story had on me. That was the first time I was so bluntly confronted by the impact of denial on the practice of medicine, and it triggered recollections of other cases I had witnessed. Thus, in a sense, it served as a catalyst for the entire venture of recapturing and compiling the following stories.

2.

DOUBLE-CROSSED

The young man who came to see me was the son of an old friend and colleague. I had not seen his father in many years but remembered him well from our time together in medical school. We had been in the same four-man study team for all six years and had been quite close. Over the years I had followed his career in Haifa, but we hadn't had much contact, other than infrequent class reunions.

Dan was like his father in his younger days—stocky, barrel-chested, with pale reddish hair, very white skin, and a rather large head. He was dressed in a well-cut business suit, which immediately caught my attention. Suits were definitely not in fashion at the time for young Israelis, who generally preferred much more casual clothes. Although not good-looking—in fact, quite the opposite—he displayed a kind of virile energy, which many women, I thought in passing, might find attractive.

It turned out that he had come to see me about his father. Years earlier he had been diagnosed with a rare kind of tumor, a lipoma, growing inside the spinal canal. Though not malignant, the growth had spread within the bony confines of the vertebral canal and was compressing the nerves serving the lower limbs, causing increasing weakness. His father had undergone surgery (the only viable treatment option), which resulted, as could have been expected, in only incomplete removal of the growth; it could not be fully excised for fear of irreparable damage to those delicate nerve filaments. With a lot of physiotherapy, he had been fine for some years, but now the tumor was growing again, causing increasing weakness, amounting to partial paralysis of his lower limbs. He was in a wheelchair. The surgeons at his hospital in Haifa had warned that a new operation would be hazardous. Another surgeon had been consulted, and he too was of the same opinion.

"My father is very unhappy with these evaluations," Dan said. "He has a lot of difficulty getting in and out the car, so he insisted that I come to Tel Aviv on my own to talk to you."

"Why me?" I asked, surprised. This was all about neurosurgery and way outside my area of knowledge, let alone expertise.

"For some reason my father seems to think you could help him more than the doctors who have so far been consulted. He claims to remember your different approach to complicated medical problems and says he would value your input. He speaks of you as his oldest friend and says he believes you will give him the best advice."

Dan's tone implied loud and clear that he did not agree with his father's wish. I can't say I blamed him. This really was way beyond the limits of my experience. I knew nothing about spinal lipomas or how they ought to be managed.

"Why didn't your father call me himself?" I asked.

"He leaves all medical arrangements to me," he replied curtly.

I remembered his father as always having a ready smile and a keen sense of humor. The son, I sensed, was dour and overly self-confident. There was also an air of controlled aggression in his demeanor, perhaps even bordering on arrogance. These were all just first impressions, but after so many years working with patients, you develop an instinct about people. And I have learned to trust my instincts.

Dan drew his father's CT films out of a handsome brown leather briefcase and handed them to me. Although I am no expert in radiology of the spine, it was immediately clear to me that the tumor was indeed tightly lodged in the spinal canal around the nerve roots and probably very difficult to approach in an operation, let alone remove. I suggested a consultation with our neurosurgeons and offered to show them the CT films first. Dan agreed but impressed upon me the importance of speed, as his father was becoming extremely agitated and wanted to know as soon as possible what could or should be done. I promised to expedite matters and get back to him quickly. I also put it to him that no self-respecting neurosurgeon would offer an opinion without first talking to his father in person and examining him. He would certainly have to bring his father to our hospital for examination as soon as I could arrange things.

That afternoon I went to see our neurosurgical team. They went over the films with their radiology consultant and discussed the case at length. The consensus was that the surgeons in Haifa had been right in their judgment, and that attempted removal of the tumor would probably cause much more immediate harm than would just leaving it in place. My only contribution was to point out that in the final analysis, the decision rested on questions relating to quality of life, given that possible cure was no longer a viable option. We had not seen the patient. We had no firsthand knowledge of how he was coping with his current degree of disability. Only he could give us the insights we needed as to his expectations and how clear in his mind were the serious risks involved in both options, including neurological deterioration, possibly ending up with paralysis and incontinence. Our chief neurosurgeon immediately offered to see the patient as soon as we could get him there. Thanking him, I went back to my office to phone Dan and ask when he could bring his father to Tel Aviv, explaining the ins and outs the neurosurgical team had discussed and all the possible ramifications.

His response took me aback. "Is all this really necessary?" he asked. "My father has been subjected to so many tests and examinations. He is simply too tired to undergo any more of them. Can't you people make up your minds without dragging him through another round of hassle? I suppose," he went on, "that we'll have to go through the whole rigamarole of medical insurance coverage, and then once that is settled we will probably have to make an appointment, which will also take months; these things always do."

Needless to say, I didn't like his tone. I had, after all, taken a lot of trouble to convene a group of very busy people for an unscheduled consultation about someone who was not even a hospital patient. Our request to see his father was more than reasonable, and instead of gratitude, this pugnacious young man was grumbling about the hassle. Still, I thought, it must be his concern for his father that was driving his aggressive attitude. I decided not to react and simply reiterated our request that he bring his father to see us as soon as possible, even the next day, if he could manage.

"And," I continued, "we're doing all this for a friend and colleague; there will be no fees or charges. So, as you really are in a hurry, we'll accommodate your father's timetable. All you need to do is to get him here, possibly even tomorrow." As I was getting a little exasperated, I asked whether I could speak to his father on the phone. I really wanted to hear from him personally, how he felt and what was foremost in his mind. Dan said he was asleep, and, in any case, he didn't want his father bothered until the situation was clearer.

I did not want to get into fresh confrontations with him, so I simply told him that was the way it was going to be if he wanted our help, and I hung up.

Two weeks went by without my hearing from them. I phoned a couple of times but only got an answering machine recording. I found this surprising since, according to the information Dan had given me, his father was supposed to be unable to leave home. I was really surprised when Dan contacted me again, about a month later. Even more astonishing was his telling me that immediately after our last talk, he had decided to take his father to New York for a consultation, returning only two days earlier.

"I wanted him to be examined by the top experts in the field," he said. "Money is no object where my father's health is concerned. I have done very well and intend to use every last penny I have, if necessary, in order to see my father restored to health."

Momentarily, I felt a sense of understanding for him; he was so obviously worried about and concerned for his father. But his abrasive manner made it difficult to remain sympathetic.

"Why didn't you let me know you had changed your mind about letting our team see your father?" I asked.

"Well, he actually did want to come to hear your opinion and even ask you to refer us to the top people in the States, but I thought you would probably not be too happy about our decision to seek advice elsewhere. You know, the old 'local guild' mentality," he answered with what could almost be described as a sneer. I was taken aback but again decided to avoid confrontation. I simply asked him what the American doctors had proposed.

It turned out that they had been to one of the best spinal surgery centers in New York. The doctors there had apparently held out reasonable hope for recovery with the aid of special innovative microsurgery. I asked to see a written report. He promised to fax it to me.

"So why are you calling?" I asked. "Can I help you with anything else?"

"Well, my father still insists that I discuss with you the American surgeons' opinion that surgery is warranted. He is rather old-fashioned and believes that his local medical colleagues are the best. In light of their unanimous opinion that surgery would be harmful, he is uneasy and very much wants to hear your opinion. Could we speak again after you've seen the reports?"

At this point I told him that before going any further I had to see his father. "If a trip to Tel Aviv is too strenuous for him, I am perfectly willing to come to Haifa and visit with him at home. For old times' sake," I said, thinking, perhaps unkindly, that Tel Aviv was closer than the United States and the effort far less formidable.

Dan attempted to persuade me to give him the benefit of my opinion based on the detailed information that he was sending me. I refused, explaining again that the decision revolved solely around his father's own assessment of his prospects if surgery failed. Without a one-on-one discussion with his father, I would not venture an opinion nor offer any further advice. Dan was not pleased with my response and ended the conversation rather sullenly, stating that he would call again after talking to his father. I considered phoning his father myself, as I found it even stranger that we still had not talked directly, that all contact had been through Dan. I decided, however, that attempting to bypass the son would cause trouble and be interpreted as interference on my part. I decided to wait and see whether Dan would contact me again.

He phoned a week later to ask me to come to Haifa. "I'll make it worth your while," he added. I didn't even bother to answer. We had been through the professional courtesy story before, but the man was determined to be unpleasant. Although annoyed, I had to force myself to ignore his manner if I wanted to try to help his father.

I took the next day off and drove to Haifa. Dan lived in a large villa on Mount Carmel overlooking the city and the bay beyond it, the panorama extending as far as the white cliffs of the Western Galilee mountain range, where they drop into the Mediterranean at the border with Lebanon. The garden surrounding the house was quite beautiful and gave the impression of being lovingly tended. The house itself, however, was ostentatious, its entrance adorned with a rather vulgar imitation of white Doric pillars. A maid let me in and showed me to a large terrace overlooking the garden and, beyond it, the sea.

A few minutes later Dan appeared. Casually dressed this time in an open sports shirt, jeans, and loafers, he seemed more relaxed in his own home than he had been in my office. Without any niceties, he immediately proceeded to warn me not to upset his father, who was very vulnerable and anxious. It was fine for me to sound him out, but I was not to discuss possible outcomes or prognoses with him present. Affording me no time to reply to this silly demand, he went off to bring his father, leaving me wondering what had happened to the resilient, cheerful young man I had known at medical school to make him so needy of his son's belligerent protectiveness.

Meanwhile, I noticed a young woman pruning the roses in the garden. As soon as Dan was gone, she came over and introduced herself. She was Rachel, Dan's wife, petite, slim, with straight, dark hair falling to her shoulders and nice brown eyes with long, soft lashes. She was pretty in an unassuming kind of way, and in her green cotton dress, she appeared to blend with the flowers in the garden beyond her. I guessed that the loving care I had sensed as I walked through the gate must be of her doing. She obviously knew why I had come, although she did not refer to the situation they were faced with, maintaining a stream of small talk until her husband returned with her father-in-law. She then brought a tray of glasses of fresh orange juice, set it down on a small glass table, and hastily retreated.

My old friend Marcus was in a wheelchair. Although I thought I had known what to expect after so many years, it was still shocking to see him in such a state. He must have been no more than fifty-five years old, but he looked at least ten years older. His hair was white, and his face seemed to have crumpled, yet he smiled as he saw me, the old smile I still remembered. I felt he was genuinely pleased to see me. I took his hand in mine and sat down next to him. As we reminisced a little, he seemed to come to life, even laughing aloud at some of the stories we recollected.

After fifteen minutes on memory lane, I took the plunge and asked him if he wished to talk to me about himself.

"Certainly," he replied with a smile. "That's what I dragged you up here for. Ask away."

"Well, Marcus, you already know that I am familiar with all the clinical facts. But what I really need, as I'm being asked for my humble non-specialist's opinion, is to get a feeling for what your own assessment of your condition is, what you are hoping for, and what concerns you have with respect to the decisions you have to make."

At this point Dan broke in. "I've already told you the whole story. Why are you putting my father through this kind of unnecessary questioning?"

He was truly getting on my nerves. Still, glancing at his father, I patiently explained once again that hearing Marcus describe in his own words what he was feeling would afford me far better insight into the problems we were dealing with and how best to render an opinion.

Dan again began to remonstrate loudly, but Marcus quietly admonished him. "Please stop treating me like a five-year-old and allow me to remain alone with Hillel. We have much to discuss."

Dan protested but finally gave in to his father and sullenly departed.

"You must excuse Dan," said Marcus apologetically. "He is my only son, and I have always spoiled him. He's always been used to getting his own way. You probably know that my wife left me soon after he was born. She left Israel after the divorce was settled, and I raised him on my own. It's always been just the two of us, and he is not used to being excluded from anything that concerns me."

I reassured him that Dan's behavior was of no consequence and that I had come to be with him and see if I could help him in any way to reach the best possible decision, realizing full well how difficult it must be for him.

"It's been a long time," he said with a rueful smile.

"It certainly has, too long by far. I'm sorry that our reunion is under such circumstances, but I did want to see you. Indeed, I needed to get a firsthand impression of what you were going through before telling your son what I thought. He is quite a character!"

"Yes, he certainly is, but underneath the gruff façade, he is really a good-hearted man trying to do his best for me," he said, seemingly used to the necessity of defending his son's rudeness.

"I got the impression that he was truly reluctant to let me see you. Why is that?"

His response was very precise. "He believes that the surgeons were to blame for the failure of the first operation ten years ago. He still mistrusts Israeli doctors. He is obsessed with the idea that we are all, unconsciously, members of a society for mutual protection. He thinks that you too are biased and will be against further surgery in the US, irrespective of the facts he gave you. That you will simply go along with the opinions of our surgeons here in Haifa, and yours in Tel Aviv, rather than acknowledging that what the Americans have to offer is far more advanced and better."

"Is that his only reason for such mistrust?" I asked.

For a moment there was silence. I realized that I had unwittingly struck a sensitive nerve.

"Rachel and Dan have no children now. They had a son. The child died four years ago. It was meningitis." Marcus shot out these staccato sentences in a stream. He stopped. There was a heavy silence between us. I waited for him to go on. He sat there nodding his head as though carrying on an internal conversation. He took a few deep breaths.

"Dan was abroad on business. The three-year-old boy was in kindergarten. Rachel had gone to Tel Aviv that morning and had arranged for him to be collected by one of the other mothers. The child suddenly developed a severe headache and started vomiting. They rushed him to hospital. He had a raging fever. Everything happened so fast. A spinal tap, intravenous massive antibiotics. Then there were convulsions, and he sank into a coma. It all happened within three hours. He died later that same evening—meningococcal meningitis, they told us, with overwhelming bloodstream infection. There was nothing more the doctors could do. They couldn't save him. And Dan could never forgive them."

Marcus was crying. I got up and put my arm around his shoulders. We sat like that in silence. Then he added in a whisper, "I am not sure that he ever forgave Rachel for not being there when it happened."

I poured us both some juice and gave him time to collect himself.

After a while I decided to break the silence. "I'm sorry to have upset you. There's really nothing worse than losing a child, a grandson. I think you've helped me understand your son's attitude very well. Thanks for that." He nodded and I went on. "Well, here I am and really happy to see you again. Let's try to make some sense of all the information and professional opinions confronting you. I'm only an internist, but I am a good listener. Maybe simply that—listening to you as you tell me how you see things—maybe that itself will help you make your decision. But as to your son's mistrust of our profession, you'll have to get around that obstacle on your own."

He rearranged himself in the chair and pointed to his legs. "Look at me—it's not so bad. Both my legs are very weak, can't bear my weight, but I do get around quite well in this contraption. As you can see, my son has spared no effort to redo the house to accommodate my Cadillac," he said, patting the armrests. "Rachel is very sweet and attentive. I navigate and manage myself in the bathroom, which Dan has equipped with the latest technological wonders. Quite amazing, really, these modern inventions."

"Do you have any pain?" I asked.

"No, not really. Just the occasional tingling or numbness, rarely some shooting pain that lasts no more than a few seconds. Believe me, if I could still walk, we wouldn't be having this conversation."

"How long have you known that your legs were getting worse?" I asked.

"I had a few good years after the first operation ten years ago. I knew some of the tumor had not been removed, but I was told that it was very slow-growing and possibly wouldn't cause more trouble for a long time. After all, apparently it took some twenty years or so to get to where it was at the time of the surgery. Right now, I'll take another twenty years quite happily. Anyway, about four years ago, I noticed these tingling sensations in both my legs. Then, about two weeks later, my left leg started giving out from under me as I tried to stand on it. They told me it could be some residual inflammation of the nerve linings in the spinal canal. A late complication of all the special radiology procedures I'd had, with dye injected into the spinal canal, or of the surgery itself. But I knew it was my tumor on the move again. Look, it's been a long time," he added. "I was walking until about four months ago. Maybe this is as bad as it will get."

I pulled up my chair close to his, saying, "Look, Marcus, we are both physicians. You know the score as well as I do—"

He stopped me midsentence, paused, and then responded, "Yes, I do, but as long as I'm in control of my bladder and bowels, that will do me fine. Imagine what failed surgery would do to that."

"Does that mean you've decided against more surgery at this point in time?" I asked, knowing he understood the implications full well.

"No, I haven't made my mind up yet. I'm fully aware of the risks, but then surgical technique is so much better these days with their lasers and microsurgery. And I'm sure the Americans are light-years ahead of us in this respect. Believe me, I think of nothing else. Perhaps they can clean out much more of it than last time. Maybe I'll be able to walk out of that hospital in New York," he added wistfully.

"Where does Dan fit into all this?" I asked.

"He's really keen. He promised me we'd walk out together, straight to Smith and Wollensky for a T-bone. If it were only up to him, I would have had the operation there two months ago. He's a doer, not one to sit around waiting. You know he could very well be right."

Rachel came in with a pitcher of iced tea. She hesitated, expecting perhaps to be asked to join us, but Marcus brusquely thanked her, indicating that he wanted us to be left on our own. Rachel immediately retired, or, more accurately, melted away. She gave a kind of ethereal impression of floating about a household to which she didn't truly belong.

What could I say? On the one hand, it was highly likely that without an operation the pace and severity of Marcus's incapacitation would only accelerate as the tumor grew and progressively narrowed the space in the spinal canal. On the other, the statistics supporting the specific surgical technique recommended by the Americans weren't very convincing, as their accumulated experience with this new method was limited. And what was Marcus's own assessment of the quality of life he would have if he were not only bound to a wheelchair but also incontinent and otherwise handicapped? Still, I could not leave my reflections unspoken. He had requested my advice and, however difficult it was for me, I thought I it was my duty to comply.

"Look, Marcus," I said. "It's clear to me that you have all the information you may require. Your reasoning is sound. You know as well as I do that statistics can get you to the point of making the decision, but once you've made it, the outcome of the individual case is really unpredictable. Seeing you here at home and listening to what you have been saying, my instinct, in your case, is to leave well enough alone. But obviously you will know how to make your decision. Whatever you decide, you can count on me to help you in anything you need."

He didn't reply. We sat in the afternoon sunshine, not talking, just thinking. After twenty minutes or so, I stood up and thanked him for letting me see him.

"No, it is I who should thank you," he said, clasping both my hands in his. "Whatever happens, I will remember your devotion and caring.

I know how difficult it must have been for you. To accept one's fate or to continue the fight regardless of consequences—these decisions are so personal, so fine-tuned to one's own needs and hopes, I know that only I can make the choice, and in the final analysis it is entirely my responsibility. I hope I don't make a mistake."

With that we parted. I also said my good-byes to Rachel, who had come into the room and was standing silently beside Marcus. As I headed for the main entrance, I found Dan waiting impatiently in the front hall.

"That certainly took a long time. Well, what do you think?" he asked in his characteristically unpleasant tone of voice.

"Your father is a very wise man, Dan. The decision is extremely difficult, but he has the entire wherewithal for making it. Whatever he decides to do, he'll need all the support he can get from his family. What he doesn't need is pressure from anyone, however well-intentioned they may be. I am confident that he will make his own decision wisely. My own recommendation is to leave well enough alone. The proffered surgery is a hazardous enterprise and could lead to severe consequences. The first rule in medicine is *Primum non nocere*, 'First and foremost, do no harm.' Nobody can tell how long your father will be able to maintain his current level of functioning. But this new surgery bears too much of a risk of leaving him fully invalided. The decision is his to make. Let him make it free of pressure."

Dan shrugged his shoulders as if to say, "I don't need your advice" and offered, again, to pay me for my services. I refused, again, without showing my anger, and departed.

Driving back to Tel Aviv, I wondered what I would do if I were Marcus and whether it had been right to tell Marcus what I thought was best. There's obviously a limit to how much you can put yourself in your patient's place. Moreover, trying to do so might be counterproductive in those frequent situations in which only detached and dispassionate reasoning is called for. On the other hand, there is so much more to being a physician than just rational decision making. We too harbor feelings, anxiety, and fear. We empathize with our patients, and we are frustrated by our inability to truly help so many of them. We feel their suffering and are fearful of increasing it through error or oversight. I had learned over the years that listening carefully to the patient would let you hear, finally, what it was that he or she wanted to hear you say. This was particularly applicable when the real story was only bad and heading for worse.

But it wasn't much help when dealing with decisions that could go either way. I thought Marcus wanted to hear me say that I too was against more surgery, and that is what I said to Dan. Yet much as I couldn't stand Dan's behavior, I could understand his approach. I had to admit that if I myself were the patient under the same circumstances, I would opt for surgery in the best hands I could find. Make or break. Probably the tension between these two opposites had fueled my anger at Dan. In a sense, he had put me over a barrel, forcing me to make a recommendation I couldn't make. Quality of life is so subjective. How can a doctor be expected to give advice in these situations?

In my day this wasn't taught in medical school. Nowadays they're trying to create more "objective" methods for assessing quality of life. The buzzword is cost-effectiveness, which is becoming an important subject in medical training programs and the current literature. Yet my feeling is that despite all the professional jargon, the bottom line in trying to gauge patients' assessments or expectations of their quality of life will remain the doctor's gut feeling.

It was late evening when I got home. The day's experience had left me tired and depressed. I really hoped Marcus would make the correct choice for himself.

Not unexpectedly, I didn't hear from Dan, so after two weeks had gone by, I phoned to find out what had been decided. Rachel answered and told me that Dan and Marcus had gone to the States again. She believed that Marcus had decided to undergo surgery. I must admit I was surprised. I had left his home feeling he was inclined to leave things be for the time being and not embark on any active intervention. I wondered whether his son had heeded my advice to let his father make up his mind without exerting any pressure on him. Somehow, in the light of my brief acquaintance with him, I doubted this. I felt sad because I really feared that surgery would be counterproductive and might cause Marcus more harm than good. I waited to hear from him or Dan. I really hoped that I had been wrong in my assessment and that surgery would effect a miracle against all odds.

They had been gone for a month, during which I phoned Rachel several times. She sounded reluctant to talk and didn't seem to know much. Perhaps, I thought, she'd been instructed not to give out any information.

Another month went by, and then one morning, upon opening the newspaper at breakfast, I saw Marcus's name in large black letters followed by an announcement of his funeral, which was to take place in Haifa the next day.

I was stunned. Although I'd feared the rapid deterioration an unsuccessful surgery might lead to, I hadn't expected Marcus to die. Colleagues who had been at medical school with us phoned me to find out what had happened and perhaps, as often happens in such cases, to ventilate their own unease when someone of their age group dies unexpectedly. But I had no information to give them.

The funeral took place in a beautiful cemetery at the foot of Mount Carmel. To my surprise, the turnout was extremely large. I had gathered from my conversation with Marcus that he had rather cut himself off from his colleagues and friends as a result of his illness and had withdrawn into a more or less monastic seclusion in the past four years. Yet here were all these mourners.

Dan stood silently, receiving the stream of people who lined up to shake his hand and express their condolences. Rachel too, in a long black dress and straw hat, talked to many of the people but somehow seemed not to fit in. There was no contact between Dan and her—no linking of arms, no exchanged comforting glances, nothing.

I approached Dan and shook his hand. I attempted to say something to him. He did not answer and looked through me. It seemed to me to go beyond his customary rudeness exacerbated by grief. The glance he gave me was full of hate and anger. Had I imagined it? What could he possibly have against me? After all, I had done my best to help his father. No, it must have been my imagination, I thought.

Then the funeral was over. I laid a stone on the earthen mound covering Marcus's grave, as is the custom here, and turned around to leave the cemetery. On the way to my car, I saw Rachel walking alone in front of me. I caught up with her and asked if she would tell me what had happened in New York. Could she describe the circumstances of Marcus's death?

At first she was reluctant to talk to me and looked furtively around to see whether Dan was anywhere in sight. Seeing that he was still busy inside the cemetery, she hurriedly told me the story.

"After you left our house, Marcus told Dan that he had decided not to have surgery and asked him to cancel the trip to New York. Dan was furious and refused to believe that his father would respect the opinion of a local 'quack,' ignoring his own thoroughly researched, scientifically grounded opinion and the recommendations of the top American surgeons. I think that the time and money Dan spent on gathering information made it impossible for him to honor Marcus's rejection of his plan. He tried to convince his father that he would walk again after surgery, that he would be able to get back to his work, that life for the two of them would be back to what it was before the illness. They would travel to places together, see the world, and do all the things that his illness had prevented them from doing."

She stopped for a minute, and I wondered whether it had occurred to her that she had said "they" would travel together and not "we." I wondered what her position in that household had been. It seemed to me that she had long ago accepted the role of an invisible, inaudible audience to the enclosed and enclosing oedipal drama.

Assuring herself that Dan was nowhere in sight, she continued. "The discussions went on and on until finally Marcus gave way." Again she stopped. Almost in a whisper she then confided, "I wonder if Marcus didn't concede simply to please Dan. I don't think he wanted to go to the States, but it was so important for Dan that he finally agreed, for his sake. Anyway, when they got there, it seems the American surgeons warned both of them repeatedly of the dangers involved. Only when assured that Marcus had taken all the consequences into account in making his decision did they proceed with the operation.

"Dan phoned me while his father was in the operating theater, almost hysterical with anxiety and fears lest the warnings had been right, alternating with hope that his father would walk out of the hospital. He would show everyone in Israel how wrong they had been. But the surgery did not go smoothly. The next thing I heard was that Marcus was paralyzed from the waist down and incontinent. Dan was beside himself with grief. Two weeks later he realized that there was nothing further that could be done for Marcus in New York and made arrangements to bring him back to Israel.

"They were supposed to come back two weeks ago, but Marcus suddenly took a turn for the worse. Infection around the bladder catheter rapidly turned into bloodstream infection. Sepsis, they called it. Despite massive antibiotics and intensive care support, Marcus's condition deteriorated rapidly. He died a week later. Dan told me that it seemed as if all the fight had gone out of him. That he truly no longer wished to live." Rachel cried quietly. "He came back in a coffin."

I asked her how Dan was taking it and whether I could do anything to help.

"You don't understand. It is you that he blames. He says you convinced his father to have the surgery. He says that it was only as a result of your visit that his father decided to go to the States. He says he was against it, and you convinced Marcus that he should take the risk. Without your intervention, according to Dan, Marcus would still be alive," she whispered.

I was dumbfounded. I could not grasp what she was saying. How could the truth be turned upside down? Undoubtedly it must have been excruciatingly painful for Dan to admit to himself that he was instrumental in his father's death, but could he really have succeeded in denying reality so completely by shifting the blame onto me? Was it possible that he really believed that our roles had been reversed? At that moment, Rachel caught sight of Dan and quickly walked away from me.

I stood in the middle of the path still in shock when Dan passed me without a glance in my direction or a word uttered.

I drove back to Tel Aviv, my head abuzz with doubts as I tried to reconstruct my last visit with Marcus in Haifa. Could it be that I hadn't made clear to Dan that I was not in favor of surgery? No, it couldn't; I remembered his hostility well when I told him my position. But could it be I had somehow intimated to Marcus my own covert feelings, that I myself would have chosen the surgery? And could it be that this was the message he'd passed on to Dan? No, that too was impossible; Rachel had given me a very clear account of how Dan had practically bulldozed his father into agreeing to surgery.

Furious though I was, I decided to write Dan a letter of condolence. It came back unopened. A few days later Rachel phoned.

"I'm calling to apologize for Dan's behavior. You must understand that blaming you is the only way he can deal with his grief and anger at failing to stem the tide of his father's illness. He is a very complicated man and is suffering deeply. Please forgive him and accept my thanks in Marcus's name for your caring and efforts on his behalf."

Rachel sounded as though she was crying. I thanked her for her call and told her that if there was anything I could ever do to help her, she need only phone.

I never saw Dan again, or Rachel. I have often wondered whether he still lived within the world of reversed truth and fallacy he had created for himself and whether perhaps he had finally stopped blaming Rachel for the death of their child. I hope, as time goes by, both of them will find a measure of peace.

3.

MEDICAL MEDLEY

I first met Lisa at a New Year's Eve party at a friend's home. She was an attractive brunette with a lively face framed by a cloud of hair that brought to mind a lion's mane. Her green dress set off a pair of bright eyes of the same color, which held my gaze as we found ourselves talking, somehow removed from the people milling about in the room. She was thirty-five years old, recently divorced, and had one child, a six-year-old daughter. She held a master's degree in mathematics and worked in the civil service.

Within minutes we had cut through the obligatory small talk and were engaged in a heated debate over Philip Roth's *Portnoy's Complaint,* which we had both recently read. Lisa disliked the portrayal of the Jewish mother and thought it a grotesque caricature. I loved the book and identified with Roth's portrayal of the New York Jewish family and especially of Sophie, the mother. Many of the episodes described seemed to have been taken directly from my own childhood in New York; the scene in the clothing store, for example, of Portnoy's humiliation when his mother refuses to buy him a bathing suit with a jock strap, jokingly asking whether his "little thing" really warranted it.

Reading that section, I'd had a clear recollection of going through a somewhat similar experience, remembered to this very day, with my own mother. I was nine years old, and we were shopping at Alexander's for new trousers. I found a pair of brown corduroys I liked and was sent off to try them on. I'll never forget the sickening embarrassment I felt when she then made me bend forward, my rear end facing her, and made sure, manually, that there was "enough room in the crotch."

Lisa had grown up in Israel and was simply unable to accept that Roth's descriptions were anything but the result of a "neurotic, warped, sex-obsessed, infantile mind." We argued on and on, ignoring the champagne, the music, and the partying going on around us. She was easy to talk to, smart and full of humor, and I found myself reluctant to leave her company and blend back into the flow of the party.

Several weeks later we happened to meet again, this time at a little coffee bar near the hospital where I often stopped for an espresso. She was alone at her table and, smiling, invited me to join her. Again our conversation flowed easily, as if we were truly longtime acquaintances. As we talked I noticed that her hands and forearms were covered with a bad rash and quite a few scratch marks.

"I see that the doctor in you also finds me interesting," she bantered, following my gaze.

"Indeed he does," I replied in the same spirit. "May I ask what happened to your skin?"

It was a strange story. She had been suffering from this recurring skin rash for the last two years and had been seen by quite a few well-known dermatologists. She had also consulted with a leading specialist in London. Not one of them had come up with a specific diagnosis or was able to suggest a solution. They had prescribed many different creams and ointments, bathing in the Dead Sea, changes in her dietary habits—all to no avail. The itching, with its attendant scratching, kept recurring, to her great distress and exasperation.

I was not in the habit of soliciting patients, but she and her story intrigued me. Though not an expert on skin problems, I would gladly try to help her, I said, if that was her wish. She phoned a few days later, and we arranged for her to come the following week. Two days before her appointment, she cancelled, saying that there had been a turn for the better, the rash had receded, and she felt she was on the mend. Somehow, I was saddened that I wasn't going to see her, but I told her I was pleased to hear she was better and wished her a full recovery.

About a month later, she called again. The rash was back—worse, in fact, than it had been, having spread to her neck and chest, the itching now unbearable. This time she came as agreed, indeed looking much worse than the first time I had seen her. Her face too was red, her arms and legs scaly, and she scratched incessantly as we talked.

"It's only dermatologists who've seen me up to now," she reminded me, "and a fat lot of good they've done me. Now I've come to see a real doctor. I hope you have more to offer than magic creams or potions," she added challengingly.

"How long has this been going on?" I asked her.

"About two years, but it comes and goes. Sometimes I'm fine for months, and then suddenly the itching and rash erupt again, again lasting months. I'm really miserable, at the end of my tether. The skin doctors have tried countless therapies. One covered my whole body with a kind of tar, another sent me to the Dead Sea for mud treatments, a third scraped the rash with a kind of spatula and then spread a pasty ointment over the whole area. It burned like hell and did absolutely no good. Yet another injected me with ACTH for weeks. I blew up like a balloon and looked horrible, but that didn't help either. I was dosed with antihistamines galore. The most annoying of all the doctors was Professor Feynman, who fancied himself a psychologist and started questioning me about my dreams. I suppose he must have thought that my condition was psychosomatic. What an idiot!" She stopped for breath.

Her words gave me pause. Decades earlier I had done my internship and residency training with one of the world's leading proponents of the mind-body connection, Dr. Johannes Juda Groen, or J. J., as we called him. A Dutchman, he had been chief of medicine at the Wilhelmina Hospital in Amsterdam, escaping in time to England in 1940, just ahead of the Nazi invasion. He had brought his psychosomatic doctrine to our university hospital in Jerusalem in the 1960s, where he was appointed professor of medicine. He was a very short man, no taller than five foot four, with a huge head covered in swept-back white hair and penetrating green eyes framed by gold-rimmed spectacles. His Hebrew was rudimentary, but mixed with accented English. He had no problem expounding his precept that many physical ailments were probably driven by major psychological mechanisms seated in the brain and affecting specific body systems through neurophysiological mechanisms.

We, the house staff, were henceforth expected to address those elements with the same zeal we had been taught to invest in our selection of medications we prescribed for our patients. Adopting this approach would undoubtedly help patients recover more rapidly and fully. This policy was to be the rule. We were not allowed to administer drugs to dilate the airways of an asthmatic during an acute attack without first trying to break the bronchial spasm by gently "talking him out of it" for at least twenty minutes. Morphine was not to be injected into the vein of a patient gasping for breath in acute heart failure without first "attempting to calm her" with soothing personal contact for at least ten minutes. Nor could cortisone be used to alleviate the cramps and blood-tinged diarrhea of active ulcerative colitis until the patient had gone through a trial of a few days of talking sessions with a personal therapist (often the professor himself), along with being restricted to a liquid diet.

All this was long before our current era of double-blind, placebo-controlled clinical trials and evidence-based therapeutics, but there were successes here and there. These J. J. had written up extensively in Dutch medical publications in the 1950s. He had even coined a new diagnostic category—"syndrome shift," he called it—describing in a major American journal a series of cases in which the patients had for years manifested sequences of recurring physical ailments affecting one body system after another. These had resolved only when emotional problems, often linked to adverse changes in life circumstances, were aired and addressed.

Over the years I came to realize how extreme J. J.'s approach had been. However, I remained committed to the school of thought that recognized the need for more attention to psychological evaluation of and intervention in supposedly "pure" physical ailments. We know very well today that so much of what crosses the office threshold of a general internist is emotional in nature. Recognizing this, I had helped quite a few patients overcome their symptoms by simply listening empathetically to their stories and being available for them whenever they needed to talk.

The man that Lisa referred to as an idiot happened to be one of Israel's most prominent dermatologists, well known and respected outside the country as well. I wondered if he hadn't been right on target but reminded myself to reserve judgment until I had more information. I told her I would like to take a closer look at the rash. Could I examine the afflicted areas? She undressed with the tired air of someone who had gone through this routine countless times before.

The rash was really quite severe, and even in places where it had healed, there were still large, bumpy welts. The skin of her arms and forearms looked particularly bad, covered with leathery, thickened patches. I noticed, however, that there was one area of skin, in the middle of her back, up between her shoulder blades, that was completely unaffected. Acting on intuition, I asked her to reach out to her back with either hand to try to scratch this area. She attempted to do so repeatedly, but even her fingertips couldn't quite reach it. It didn't take much more deduction on my part to confirm my feeling that Professor Feynman had been absolutely right. There was no skin damage, no rash, where there could be no scratching.

We were dealing, then, with neurodermatitis, better known today as PSP, short for pathologic skin picking. This chronic condition is included by psychiatrists in the group of impulse control disorders. Its main psychological feature is the person's inability to resist an impulse or temptation to perform an act harmful to oneself. The individual suffers increasing inner tension, which triggers the act itself, followed by relief, or even a sense of gratification. In some patients PSP may express itself as an obsessive-compulsive disorder. These patients tend to repeat stereotyped intentional behavior as a means of alleviating anxiety or distress. In PSP the initiating sense of itching and repeated scratching inevitably produce inflammation in any area of previously healthy skin. The scratch-itch cycle sets in, fueled by periods of emotional stress and decreasing in severity during calmer times. All this tied in very well with Lisa's reported intermittent improvements between renewed attacks.

Treatment of PSP consists of a variety of stress management techniques combined with relatively simple physical routines such as tepid baths or showers several times a week and a variety of soothing skin creams. In most cases these joint measures afford a certain degree of control, and only in severe cases of recalcitrant inflammation is the use of potent cortisone creams recommended. New methods nowadays include music therapy and biofeedback techniques, all aimed at controlling the compulsive need to scratch. It is, however, notoriously difficult to cure without truly breaking the scratch-itch cycle by addressing the underlying emotional problems and achieving some form of resolution.

But how was I to explain all this to Lisa without being relegated to the status of another "idiot" in company with Professor Feynman? If I were to overcome this intelligent woman's resistance, I needed to find the right approach. I felt that the personal relationship we had developed might engender more trust, the most important factor in this kind of treatment. I knew I was venturing into territory beyond my expertise, but I had a strong feeling, perhaps naïve, that by appealing to her logical way of thinking, I could get her to relinquish the scratching itself without having to resort to psychotherapy. Choosing my words carefully, I explained why Professor Feynman might actually be right.

"I know you won't like the diagnosis any more than before, but I hope you'll not reject it out of hand without giving me the chance to try to convince you of its validity. In my opinion, you are suffering from a condition we call neurodermatitis." Lisa looked blank. She was obviously not familiar with the term. "Neurodermatitis is a self-inflicted disorder. You yourself actually cause the rash by scratching; your skin reacts to the scratching by producing an itch, which in turn causes you to scratch again, with subsequent inflammation and chronic thickening of the skin. The reasons for the problem are indeed emotional, but we might be able to break the cycle if you can accept what I have just told you."

I watched Lisa closely as I was speaking. She was clearly disappointed, on the verge of tears. This was not what she had hoped to hear. She had been expecting a cure, a drug, a cream, an injection, something tangibly physical, not a litany of psychological mumbo jumbo. I could see her thinking that I was one more incompetent in the series of so-called healers that had so disappointed her thus far.

"Will you let me show you something that might convince you of the truth of what I've told you?" I asked.

She nodded. Giving her a hand mirror, I stood her with her back to the wall mirror in my office. I asked her to lift her shirt again and carefully scrutinize the reflection of her bare skin. Pointing to the one clear area in the center of her back, I asked her if she could think of any reason why this patch of skin had remained unaffected. Lisa studied her back silently for a few minutes and then turned to me in surprise.

"Are you telling me that this is the only place on my body that I can't reach with my hands and therefore can't scratch?"

"I'm not telling you anything. It is you yourself who has just provided a very reasonable explanation for the phenomenon," I said. "I know it's not much to go on, but it's a small indication that what you have is indeed neurodermatitis. Please think about it. If you decide you'd like to try to work on it with me, I'll gladly put together a plan that we could implement together. We might be able to break the cycle and allow the skin to regain its health."

Lisa didn't say a thing. Then, without a word, she got up and walked out of the office. Very sadly, I thought that I had seen the last of her.

Leaving for home an hour later, I saw Lisa sitting in her car outside my office. I walked up to her and asked if she was all right. She didn't answer. I opened her car door and sat down beside her. After a long moment of silence, without turning toward me, she said glumly, "I think you're right. The clear patch on my back doesn't make sense any other way. I want to try to break the cycle. Help me."

I knew that in assenting I would be assuming a serious responsibility. I was neither a psychiatrist nor a psychologist. However, I had the strong feeling that I had broken the ice with Lisa, perhaps by virtue of what I construed as the beginning of a real personal relationship. If I were to refer her elsewhere, even to a specialist better equipped to deal with such ailments, the momentum gained might be lost. Lisa could very well change her mind and revert to her previous pattern of denial and rejection. Without further deliberation I told her I would help her to the best of my ability, with the condition that she allow me to bring in a psychiatrist colleague if necessary. She was somewhat reluctant but, to my delight, eventually agreed.

The cycle-breaking plan was simple—we'd schedule regular meetings to review the previous week's events at home, at the office, and specifically about the itch. I also prescribed a mild skin softener for regular use and a weak cortisone cream to be applied if the itch became severe. At my request she also made time available for a daily one-hour physical fitness session.

Before long I came to know Lisa better and found myself looking forward to our weekly meetings. In the course of our long chats, I also learned of her unhappy marriage. She had married far too young, and for all the wrong reasons, as she put it.

"He was good-looking, lots of fun, a great dancer and sports companion. All of which wore off quite quickly as daily life and baby care took over." She found out about his infidelities about a year into the marriage, and despite the initial blow to her ego, she discovered, much to her surprise, that she really didn't care that much. The marriage continued out of inertia. They had very little in common, and conversation at home dwindled to the inane. A few years later, she got up one morning and announced at breakfast that she wanted a divorce. Her husband didn't object and everything proceeded very amicably.

"As a matter of fact, he is much nicer now as a friend than he was as a husband," she said laughingly.

But I could sense sadness and loneliness behind the gay laughter. She had built a good life for herself, raising her daughter on her own as well as maintaining a successful career in database management in the government social services branch. There was almost no input from the father to his little girl's upbringing.

"It isn't that he doesn't love her," Lisa said. "He does, very much. But he just isn't the type to devote any attention to anyone who doesn't share his own immediate interests. You must have met such people—essentially nice, but supremely self-centered and completely unaware of the fact."

Lisa's story wasn't particularly unique. I had heard many such sagas before, but there was something about her personality that made it different. It may have been the timbre of her voice, deep and modulated, or her attractive looks and spirited, argumentative way of speaking. Perhaps it was the way her entire face lit up when she laughed, a full, joyful kind of laugh that invited you to share the humor of a situation. It may have been a sense of mutual attraction between us. Or all of these combined. I found myself thinking of her as a woman, but immediately realized I had better be very careful if our friendship were to remain within the appropriate limits.

Our weekly talks continued, and I was truly astounded when, within a month, the angry red excoriations were gone, leaving only the areas of thickening where the worst damage had been done. By the end of three months, the rash had virtually cleared up, and Lisa had completely stopped fingering her skin. She always carried some cortisone cream in her bag, applying it the moment she felt the slightest itch, even that of a mosquito bite. This, but mostly her trust in me, I felt, had enabled her to regain control and stop the scratching. The improvement was amazing, and Lisa was wildly happy. I too was elated, as would be any doctor who manages to help a patient overcome a severe chronic affliction. But sadness was there too as I realized I would soon be losing contact with her. And indeed, when Lisa's skin ailment had resolved, our meetings ended.

Then, about two years later and out of the blue, Lisa was back in my office. She looked well. Her skin was glowing, and even the thickened patches on her forearms had cleared up. She told me that she had fallen in love with the man of her dreams and was about to remarry. Her little daughter adored him, and she thought they would be very happy together.

"So what brings you back to see me?" I asked with a smile.

"Well, seeing as you did such a great job with my skin, I thought you might be able to help me with something else that's bothering me. I never talked to you about this before. I must have been too embarrassed at the time we met. You see, I have been constipated most of my life. It started when I was a little girl. It runs in our family. I have been on laxatives for years. Lately I've been using a special Indian tea, but it gives me the runs every time I drink it. Now that I am getting married again, I would really like to stop the unpleasant morning toilet ritual. I thought you might be able to suggest some other medication I could use in order to regulate my bowel movements, without all the associated unpleasantness."

"I'm amazed you never told me about this problem during all those months we were working together. Why didn't you?" I asked. Obviously, I had repeatedly and carefully documented Lisa's medical history throughout the period we spent working on her skin problem. She had not mentioned any previous illnesses or other present disorders.

"It just never occurred to me it was relevant. Besides, it's always been so much a part of my life that I never viewed it as a disorder. It's just normal for me to take a laxative every day. I have been doing so for as many years as I can remember."

Ordinarily, a patient who starts developing constipation, with no previous history of this nature, would merit a full diagnostic workup, including colonoscopy, to rule out the possibility of organic disease. But this was not the case with Lisa. I had learned a lot about her over the time we had spent dealing with her skin. Moreover, an ailment that had been present since childhood and not changed in pattern over thirty years was not very likely to be of any serious physical nature.

"Are you able to recall, more or less, when your preoccupation with the regularity of your bowel movements first manifested itself?" I asked.

"Well, not exactly, but I do know it had a lot to do with my father's beliefs and habits," she replied. "I remember, even as a young child, his repeatedly saying, 'You must have a bowel movement every day; it's very important that you do, because it is very unhealthy not to.' He himself had suffered from constipation all his life, having become so addicted to prune juice that he was unable to travel away from home without making sure there would be adequate supplies along the way. He used to bring me a large glass of the dark brown potion every morning. I hated it but always drank it." Lisa shuddered at the memory. "I adored my father and didn't want to upset him."

"What happened when you grew up?" I asked.

"For quite a few years, I had periods of reasonably regular bowel movements, but then, particularly in my early teens, they really became few and far between. The only way I could relieve myself was by using laxatives. My parents took me to doctors all over Europe, but none could help. Some called it a nervous bowel and recommended a variety of different diets. Some recommended yoga. One doctor even suggested I adopt a certain acrobatic crouching position on the toilet seat to ease the process. That just brought on pain down there, which turned out to be caused by hemorrhoids, which I never knew I had. The turning point was about a year ago, when I found this marvelous Indian tea that is completely natural. I take it every night before going to bed, knowing I'll be on schedule the next day. The only trouble is that I can't seem to get the dose right. Very often I have to deal with a rush of watery productions in the morning hours, and I really don't want this to continue. You know, I'll be sharing the bathroom with a new husband pretty soon."

I realized that what Lisa was describing in such plastic detail was yet another psychophysical disorder, chronic laxative abuse. Once again, I thought that the right way to help her was by appealing to her logical way of thinking. It might seem strange that a person with such neurotic manifestations could also be so coolly rational, yet that was the way she dealt with the world. She kept her fears and inner conflicts well stowed away in the recesses of her mind and remained supremely cerebral and organized externally. Again, I thought the way to convince her that she could overcome her problem would be through a change in her perception of her own body.

"Lisa," I asked, "what do you think would happen if you did not have a bowel movement every morning?"

"I don't have to guess. I know what happens. I have been through it so often. First of all, I get bloated. Then I feel heavy; my stomach feels distended. Also my clothes get tight on me," she added with a sheepish smile.

"Oh," I responded, "is it that you're worried about putting on weight as a result of your constipation?" It was fairly common knowledge that for many people, particularly women with this problem, weight gain was a primary concern.

"Well, naturally, that too," Lisa admitted.

I then launched into my standard catechism of calories eaten versus calories burned in daily activities and exercise as the secret of maintaining a desired weight. Lisa looked unconvinced.

I next drew out a sheet of paper and began drawing a graph. Lisa craned her head to see what I was doing. I didn't know if this was going to work, but I was going to give it a try.

"Take a look, Lisa, what do you see?"

"Well, I see the days of the week and the numbers that are marked next to them."

I explained that the numbers were the weight of the stool that an average human being excreted daily. I then drew a second graph showing the weight of the stool if excreted every second day and then every third and so on. I explained to Lisa that some people only "go" once in four days or more; nonetheless, the weight of the stool in the end will average out, with no difference between those who go regularly daily and those who only go twice a week. The only difference would be the amount of water in the stools. The longer the intervals, the drier (and possibly lighter) the product, but water, as she certainly knew, had nothing to do with real body weight. Therefore, I continued my sermon, that contrary to common belief, one does not gain weight if one's bowel movements occur less frequently than once a day

Lisa still seemed unconvinced. "Are you telling me it's normal to have bowel movements only once or twice a week?"

"'Normal' is not a term I use," I explained. "What is normal for one person may be abnormal for another. I am saying it won't do you any harm if you do not have a bowel movement every day or even every two or three days or more."

Lisa sat, slowly digesting my words. Again, she seemed reluctant to accept them, but I thought it was extremely important she shake off her old misconceptions. The benefit would be physical too—she'd give her intestines time to slowly recover from the sluggishness induced by years of using laxatives.

"Look," I said, "why don't we try the following routine? Expect to have a bowel movement twice a week, and do not attempt to force it until you absolutely feel the need to go. In other words, I do not want you to go to the toilet unless you feel an urgent need. Now that you know that it's 'normal,' as you put it, try to relax about it and come back to me in a week's time."

I also prescribed a locally acting, bulk stool softener for her to use during the period in which she would gradually withdraw from her reliance on fluid laxatives. Lisa agreed and I suggested that she busy herself with the wedding arrangements and forget to keep count of the days.

A week later, Lisa was back again. She was still tense but reported that she had not had to wait a week. Her bowels had worked on the fourth day. It was the first time in years that she had not used a laxative. She complained that it had been very painful, so I changed her softening prescription and asked her to return two weeks later.

This time she seemed more relaxed and reported that she had only had to wait three days. We continued in this way for several more visits, and then I suggested that she should stop coming, asking instead that she phone me from time to time just to tell me how she was doing.

I received Lisa's wedding invitation a few months later. I did not really want to renew social contacts with her, but she still intrigued me. Besides, I wanted to assure myself that I had done the right thing in treating her myself instead of referring her to a psychiatrist. The wedding was a grand affair, and Lisa looked ravishing in white. She seemed happy to see me. She whispered that she felt free for the first time. With my help, she said, she had managed to beat her body.

A few months later, she phoned just to say hello.

"You know," she said, "the other day I suddenly realized that I no longer keep count of my bowel movements and I don't even know how often I have them. Isn't it strange? I no longer care. It used to be so important to me, and now I don't even remember."

I suppose it is only natural to feel pride in one's professional successes, and I remember feeling extremely pleased with myself at the time. I did not really question the ease with which Lisa's severe symptoms were cured, although it did cross my mind that her real inner problems had not really been addressed. Things may have been just too easy. However, in the afterglow of a successful strategy, I suppose I must have pushed aside any such doubts and celebrated along with Lisa what seemed to be a complete recovery.

She kept in touch sporadically, happy in her marriage, her little girl doing fine, her career flourishing, and her health good. Then one day she phoned to let me know that her husband had received a very attractive job offer in Boston and that they were leaving within the next few weeks.

"You don't sound too happy about it," I said.

"I don't really like changes. I'm one of those people who likes to hang on to established routines. I feel more secure that way. New places, new people, new cultures—it kind of scares me. Still, I'm sure I'll get used to it. After all, America has so much to offer, and it will be great for Daphne, my little girl. She will learn a new language, meet new children, and broaden her horizons. At her age, settling in should be relatively easy and very rewarding later on in life."

Lisa rattled all this off rather breathlessly. I felt she was making an effort to remain cheerful. "How long will you be gone?" I asked.

"We are planning on two years to begin with, but like all others who have gone before us, I suppose it might turn into a much longer affair."

I found it difficult to reassure Lisa with the usual bland remarks because I had an uneasy feeling that this move was not good for her. Despite the good show she was putting up, she was clearly still deeply immersed in the process of dealing with her emotional makeup. Wouldn't this major change of every aspect of her life impede the progress she had made so far? But what could I say? I was, after all, only her doctor, and although we had been friends, it was not my place to give advice of this kind. I told Lisa that if she ever needed to talk, I was always at her disposal and would be glad to hear from her. We said good-bye on the phone, and a few days later, I heard from mutual friends that she was gone.

Months went by and I did not hear from Lisa. I assumed all was well and that she had settled down in her new surroundings. Then one morning I was surprised to find her waiting in my office.

"Please forgive me for barging in without an appointment, but I simply had to see you. I arrived last night and am going back the day after tomorrow. My only reason for this trip is to get some more good advice from you."

Lisa's voice had that breathless quality that I had come to know, which always signified intense internal turmoil. She looked pale and wan. The rosy, healthy glow that she had had at her wedding had disappeared. Her skin looked fine, so the rash hadn't reappeared. Nevertheless, she was very tense and restless.

I invited her to share my morning coffee, and she seemed to relax a little. I asked her about her little girl, her husband, Boston. Daphne was doing fine and had adjusted very quickly to the States. Her husband was very happy in his new job. Lisa had found interesting work too and was considering enrolling in a graduate student program, perhaps even working toward her PhD.

"So what brings you to Israel for such a short time?" I asked.

"I've been getting terrible headaches. You can't imagine the pain in my head; it's driving me crazy, and I can't go on living like this." Lisa twisted her hands distractedly. She was more upset and distraught than I had ever seen her before.

"When did they start?" I asked.

"Well, about a month after our arrival in Boston, I began getting these unbelievably bad headaches. I have never had headaches before. I thought they would go away, but they didn't. They just got worse and worse. I swallowed every kind of over-the-counter pain-killer. Nothing worked, so finally I went to a doctor so that he could prescribe something stronger. The doctor asked me to describe my symptoms. I told him that the headaches were generally located on one half of my head, usually concentrated around one eye, almost always accompanied by a bad bout of nausea, and lasted around three days." Lisa stopped for breath.

"How often were you getting these headaches?"

"At least once a week."

"What did the doctor tell you?" I asked, although I was sure I already knew the answer from Lisa's description of her symptoms.

"He said I was suffering from migraines. He prescribed a new drug called Imitrex, which I should take as soon as I felt the onset of the headache. He said it would alleviate the pain. He also suggested I start taking Inderal every day to prevent the attacks. I faithfully followed all his suggestions, but nothing helped. I went back to him a few weeks later. He increased the dose of the beta-blocker, but that didn't help either. So I changed doctors. I went to a highly recommended neurologist, but he too couldn't help me. He agreed with the first doctor's diagnosis and told me to try the same drugs again. It was then that I became convinced that both of them were wrong and decided to make the trip home to see you." Lisa looked me in the eye, took a deep breath, and said, "You have always helped me in the past, you have been honest with me, and you are the only doctor I trust."

There was just one question I had to ask Lisa, although I knew the answer in advance.

"Did you tell either doctor about your past skin disorder experience?"

"No. How strange that you should ask me such a question."

"Bear with me, Lisa, I need the information. Did you tell them about your constipation problems of the past?"

"No, I did not."

It was then and there that I realized I had been wrong to treat Lisa in the first place. Clearly, I should have referred her, as good medical practice required, to a psychotherapist the moment I realized that her disorder was psychophysical, persistent, and recurring in changing forms. Was it pride and perhaps the subliminal wish to keep her as my patient because I was attracted to her? I saw all this quite clearly now. Not only had I failed to cure Lisa in helping her overcome her symptoms, but I had actually caused her to switch over time to other physical expressions of her deep anxieties. What Lisa had described to the American physicians were indeed clearly symptoms of migraine headaches. But had these doctors known about her previous history, they would probably have suspected that the lack of effect of the drugs they had prescribed indicated a psychologically driven, migraine-mimicking headache syndrome.

My training days with J. J. Groen came flooding back to me. It hit me that Lisa was manifesting precisely what he had defined as a syndrome shift. I was furious with myself for not having thought of it sooner. And Lisa herself—how could anyone so intelligent fail to see the thread connecting all her ailments, past and present? The only explanation, I surmised, was a consistent denial of a deep-seated problem. Such denial would explain why she had withheld the information from all the doctors who had treated her.

How was I to explain to her that she now needed specialized professional help and that I was not qualified to undertake any further treatment of her condition? She had come to rely on me, to the extent of flying over from the States just for this consultation. How would she react to the suggestion that someone else must take over her treatment? And was it really a psychiatrist that Lisa needed? After all, she was not psychotic nor in need of medication but rather a victim of neurosis, which calls for a good listener. Could I, after all, be that listener? Could I perhaps be the one to get Lisa to look into herself, to discover the sources of her anxiety? But then, immediately realizing the foolishness of these thoughts, I dismissed the idea of any further involvement on my part. What Lisa needed, in my view, was psychotherapy, and I was simply not qualified. I had to let go of Lisa, and she had to let go of me. There was no other way to get her to begin the journey into herself.

Lisa was troubled by my silence. "Tell me what's wrong with me," she demanded.

There was nothing I could do but to try to explain my perceptions to Lisa. It wasn't going to be easy. There were obviously well-established defense barricades that Lisa had erected over a long period, probably throughout her entire life. Was it wise for me to attempt to shake them? Should I say something soothing and attempt to convince her to see a psychotherapist without going into any detail? In the end I decided to talk to her frankly, hoping she would be able to handle it just as she had in our previous encounters.

"Look, Lisa, I could possibly 'cure' your headaches, just as we managed to 'cure' your other illnesses in the past, but you will only develop other symptoms instead. Of course, the symptoms are real, and your body is really acting up, but it's your soul that is giving your body a beating. It's your soul that is camouflaging its distress with red-herring physical ailments. You must believe me when I tell you that you really must deal with the basic psychological disorder that keeps surfacing in the forms of your physical illnesses. I am to blame for not realizing earlier on that this is what we should have done all along. Do you remember the mirror we held up to your back the first time you came to see me? In a sense that is what you must do now. You must attempt to look beyond your body's signals of distress to places you have not so far been able to observe. For this we need professional help. I would like to recommend someone whom I trust and believe could help do just this."

I deliberately talked of "we" and "us" so that Lisa would not feel that I was abandoning her. "If you follow my advice, I believe we can beat not only the symptoms but this time also get to the root of it all."

Lisa did not respond. She sat there frozen, no expression on her face. Then she suddenly jumped up, turned on me ferociously, and told me I must be mad suggesting that her ailments weren't real.

"After all I have been through, are you suggesting that my headaches are imaginary? If you had experienced the pain I feel, you would realize how ridiculous everything you have just said is. I don't need a psychiatrist. I need a competent doctor who can discover the cause of my terrible headaches. I obviously made a mistake thinking you could help me."

She stormed out of my office. I followed her and tried to talk to her, but she wouldn't listen and hastily left the building.

I felt terrible. I had botched it completely. Should I have handled it in a different way? Perhaps less directly, less honestly? I thought of contacting her husband in Boston but immediately realized I couldn't without breaking the confidentiality of our talks.

I worried about it constantly over the following weeks, feeling that I had let her down badly. Then one morning she called.

"I want to apologize for my unbelievably rude outburst in your office. You have helped me so much in the past, and I cannot forgive myself for the way I have behaved."

"I am so happy to hear from you, Lisa. Please don't apologize; I realize you must have been under great strain. Where are you calling from?" I asked, thinking that she must be back in the States.

"Actually, I am still here in Israel. I needed to be alone to think things out. My husband is very understanding and has encouraged me to stay for as long as needed. I would like to take you up on your offer to recommend a psychotherapist. I won't be able to start any form of therapy right away, as I have to get back to Boston. I have been away too long as it is. But I do want to get some idea of what is involved. I may even try to get help in Boston. I cannot make any decisions right now—I'm still too confused—but I would like more information at this stage." Lisa spoke quietly and less breathlessly than usual. She sounded resigned.

I recommended a psychologist I knew and respected and asked if she wanted me to be present at the first meeting. She said no, that she thought she could stand on her own two feet now without the need of a crutch. She promised to call me from time to time to let me know how she was doing and said a muted good-bye.

About six weeks later, I was contacted by Dr. Rosenthal, the psychologist I had recommended. He inquired about some details of Lisa's medical history and then asked me whether I would agree to a meeting with Lisa and him in my office.

I was stunned. The relationship between a psychotherapist and his patient is highly personal and private, and I had never been asked to participate in a joint session of this kind before. Was it not ethically improper? I asked.

Dr. Rosenthal understood my concern.

"It certainly is unorthodox, but in my opinion your involvement at this stage is in Lisa's interest, indeed perhaps critical to the success of her treatment," he said. "You must know that to her you are more than just her doctor."

He did not elaborate further. With some misgivings, I agreed.

A few days later, they came to my office. Lisa looked washed-out but smiled and told me that she herself had insisted on this three-sided meeting. "I hope you won't feel uncomfortable, but I wanted you to witness firsthand how I am progressing with the psychotherapy," she said.

It now transpired that with Dr. Rosenthal's help she had managed to open up a painful subject that she had not been able to confront until now. At a very early age, it turned out, Lisa had developed a father fixation. I had, in fact, noticed that she repeatedly mentioned him, not only in describing the prune juice episode, but in practically all our talks. I had not attached any special significance to this mannerism. My colleague, however, did and, upon probing, managed after several sessions to uncover one major source of Lisa's anxieties and suffering.

Her father had always been the center of her universe. She adored him, phoned him three or four times a day about every small detail of her life, and shared all her joys and troubles with him. He, in turn, encouraged this close, some might say pathological, relationship to the exclusion of his wife, Lisa's mother, who was resentful at constantly being left out of this closed association. This had been going on for years and might even, Lisa candidly admitted, have wrecked her marriage, since no mere mortal of a husband could have competed with the demigod male image she had created. Perhaps she had even subconsciously chosen a weak husband who would pose no threat to the relationship with her father.

Then one day, without any warning signs, her father had a heart attack. He was a healthy man, had never suffered any kind of ailment, and so the shock was complete. Lisa rode in the ambulance with him. It was the most frightening moment of her life. Her father was rushed into the emergency ward while Lisa remained outside, in total shock. The doctor in charge came out and asked her permission to administer a new experimental drug that he said would ameliorate the blood-flow blockage immediately. Lisa hesitated. The doctor told her that in 90 percent of cases, this drug worked wonders. If it were his father, he would administer the drug unhesitatingly. There was no time to lose, he said. Without consulting her mother, Lisa gave her permission. The drug was administered. Within minutes her father was dead. All the doctors could say was that unfortunately he had been among the minute fraction of patients who responded badly to the new treatment.

"Had I refused permission, my father would still be alive today," Lisa said. "I am directly responsible for my father's death. I have to live with that for the rest of my life. There isn't a day that goes past without me reliving that one moment when I said yes and killed my father."

Lisa cried and shook uncontrollably. I started to get up and go to her, but my colleague made a sign for me to stay in my seat. I waited for her to tell me why she had wanted me to participate in this session, but nothing more was said. After a long while she calmed down. Lisa had obviously been through this catharsis before with my colleague, but the intensity of the pain did not seem to have diminished.

And then she was gone. It was almost two years before I heard from her again. She and her husband and daughter had moved back to Israel, and she was back at her old job. She had undergone regular therapy in the States for over a year, and although she didn't feel that she was cured, she was much happier and at peace now. She still had the occasional periods of constipation, but far less severe. Her skin remained clear, and the headaches were gone.

She thanked me again for helping her realize that the problem was within her and could only be helped by hard work over a long period.

"I have finally learned to walk alone and no longer go to doctors—and I don't even need sessions with psychologists. I think I owe this newfound independence to you. I am truly grateful for everything you have done for me over the years. I realize, of course, that my problems have not vanished, but I now feel able to deal with them without seeking outside support. I sometimes get scared and am tempted to call you, but then I control the itch and get on with my life. It seems to work," she said wryly.

I have not seen her for some years now, and I actually miss her. Every doctor has some patients with whom he forms a special kind of relationship, but Lisa was more than just a patient. I always think of her with warmth and, despite the happy end, some indefinable sense of sadness.

4.

MULTIPLE VEILS

The day I first met Bella was one of the hottest days that I can remember, with temperatures at midday running about 103. A hot, dust-filled wind blew from the east, known colloquially as a *khamsin*, from the Arabic word for fifty. Tradition has it that there are fifty such days a year, with hot, parching winds blowing in from the desert. The Quonset huts—previously British army barracks, now housing the hospital wards—were sweltering. Airconditioners were a thing of the future, and only a few rickety ceiling fans slowly revolved, uselessly emitting a monotonous creaking sound that was driving me round the bend. Following the standing order of our ward chief, Dr. Ezra Zohar, the nurses had hung water-drenched sheets across all the open windows, supposedly to cool the interior through the evaporation. The sheets dried out almost as fast as they were hung, making virtually no dent in the extreme discomfort of patients and staff alike.

Dr. Zohar was a real climate freak. He was a regular army man, as were many of our senior medical staff members. The hospital had only recently been decommissioned from its military status. It had been a British rear-echelon medical facility backing up the North African front in World War II and was taken over by the Israelis when the British withdrew In 1948.

Dr. Zohar was the head of the medical corps stress physiology team, and he was one of the few at that time who totally discredited leftover British army traditions that dictated soldiers be trained for desert conditions by "learning" to do with only minimal amounts of water, one canteen a day.

He'd proved his concept of liberal water intake by conducting one of the first controlled clinical trials to be done in Israel. The physiological responses and performance of military tasks by two groups of officer cadets were compared during a three-week march from Metulla in the far north to Eilat in the very far south. The cadets marched some nine hundred kilometers at about forty a day. One group had unlimited access to drinking water while the other drank only the traditional one canteen daily. Needless to say, the data were overwhelmingly in favor of the liberal approach, by all performance variables measured. From that day on, free access to drinking water became standard procedure in our army, Dr. Zohar's contribution to posterity.

But I digress. To get back to that hot day when I first met Bella.

I had been on my feet since seven o'clock that morning and had stepped into my office to catch my breath and change my soaking hospital coat (Dr. Zohar frowned upon undershirts or T-shirts as hindering efficient sweat evaporation, natural cooling, and, hence, performance). When a very firm knock sounded at the door, I considered not answering. The knock became more insistent. My level of irritation climbed a notch. "Come in," I barked.

The intruder was a stately lady, sixty-five or so, who introduced herself rather grandly as Bella and then stared at me expectantly, as though she had just bestowed an honor on me. I couldn't quite place her, despite a vague notion of having perhaps seen her around the hospital campus on some occasion. She was quite tall with a full figure and faded blonde, permed hair that merged seamlessly with her clothes of indeterminate color. She carried a large canvas bag, which she clutched tightly. The only things noticeable in her otherwise colorless appearance were her deep blue eyes, which at that moment were staring at me imperiously.

"I am Bella," she repeated insistently.

I must have looked as confused as I felt.

"Dr. Newman talked to you about me yesterday, and you agreed to see me today at two p.m. It is now exactly two p.m. I am never late for a meeting."

Now I remembered. Dr. Newman, our gastroenterologist, had phoned a week earlier and asked me to see a patient who'd been referred to him by Professor Neufeld, our chief cardiologist. Dr. Newman had seen her, ordered a series of X-rays, and found nothing wrong. "She's quite a character, doesn't really know what we want of her," he'd said. "Be patient and empathic; you know she works for Neufeld."

With everything that had been happening that morning on the ward, I had completely forgotten the appointment. I apologized to the lady and asked her to sit down.

Her Hebrew accent was clearly American, typically New York, to my accustomed ear. By way of introduction, she immediately pointed out that she was a volunteer in Neufeld's departmental office, working as some sort of personal assistant cum English language letter writer and secretary. Moreover, she added, it was she who did all the English corrections and editing of the many manuscripts submitted by the cardiology staff to medical journals.

"Believe me," she said, "if not for my input, not a single paper would be accepted. Their English is abominable. Don't they have schools in this country?"

Neufeld was not a man to be trifled with, being one of the more prominent and influential figures on our campus, so I put on my warmest demeanor and plunged right in with my "What can I do for you?"

It turned out that although she felt fine, Neufeld had suggested she do some routine tests, "as should all people at her age." She'd agreed, humoring her boss. "But I knew exactly what the tests would show. I've had this slight anemia for years. My doctors in New York told me it was there way back in 1958. They also found that my ESR was high, something that's still that way whenever it is checked. They always get excited about it but never find anything to explain it," she said nonchalantly.

The ESR (erythrocyte sedimentation rate) was a blood test in common use in those days. Although not specific for a particular diagnosis, if it was too fast, it was often taken as an indication of some underlying condition, perhaps of an inflammatory nature but also possibly malignant. What made it unreliable was that any minor illness, such as the common cold or other respiratory tract viral infection in the preceding days, could make it go pretty high. Doctors in those days were split into two camps, the ESR believers and the debunkers. Confronted by a fast ESR, the former would launch an intensive hunt for an underlying diagnosis, subjecting the patient to myriad blood tests, X-rays, and expert consultations. The latter would adopt a conservative approach, allowing some time to elapse, repeating the test to make sure the ESR hadn't, in the interim, gone down on its own.

"Whatever else happens, young man," she said, glaring at me, her blue eyes flashing, "you can be sure of one thing: no one is going to stick any more needles or tubes into me. I've had it, big time. Like I said, these tests have been out of kilter for a very long time, but I'm still very much here, aren't I?"

At their boss's behest, the doctors in the cardiology department had put her through a battery of blood tests, which, sure enough, had demonstrated her long-standing anemia and fast ESR. Being unable to relate these findings to any problem related to her heart, they referred her to the hematologists. Further tests were done, again shedding no new light on the problem. The hematologists in turn referred her to the gastroenterologists, who ordered X-rays of her esophagus and stomach. They too found nothing wrong. Now it was my turn, as a general internist, to be asked whether I would assist.

"How can I help you?" I asked again.

"You probably can't. None of the others did. But I wouldn't worry about it, if I were you," she said graciously, as though consoling me in advance for my certain failure.

"Well, tell me anyway, and let me try," I responded, thinking that this was all I needed on that particularly unbearable day.

"Actually, since starting all these tests, I haven't been feeling as well as before," she said matter-of-factly. "Just run down, more easily tired than some weeks ago. But I'm sure it's only this damned anemia, which sometimes gets me down. I don't know what everyone is so excited about. It's probably nothing at all. I wouldn't have come to you, but Professor Neufeld insisted. The poor man got quite agitated and said he wouldn't let me come to work unless I agreed to see you. I told him you wouldn't be able to do any better than the others, but he was adamant, so here I am."

Hearing Professor Neufeld, the all-powerful despotic chief of cardiology, referred to as "the poor man" left me nearly speechless.

"Well, young man, aren't you going to get going?"

"You haven't given me a chance yet," I said. "Why don't you tell me about yourself so that I can get to know you a little better?"

By now it had probably become a question of ego too. I was young, and the opportunity of cracking a case that others had failed to diagnose made my adrenaline flow. I forgot about the heat and how tired I was and began the process of documenting her medical history. She wasn't very cooperative to begin with, but as we talked she loosened up a little, and the person behind the faded blonde shell began to emerge.

"You're originally from the States, aren't you?" I asked. "I also come from there."

She raised her eyebrows in surprise. "Are you American too? You seem to be the typical sabra." *Sabra* is Hebrew for cactus—prickly on the outside but sweet on the inside—which is supposed to characterize Israelis born in Israel.

I explained that indeed I was a sabra but born to American parents living in Palestine at the time. However, I had been raised as a boy in New York, returning to Israel when I was ten years old. I suggested we talk in English, thinking it might make her more comfortable.

"No, that is totally unnecessary. I am one hundred percent Israeli now, and my Hebrew is perfect. It's been a good twenty-five years, after all. I only go back to the States once every two or three years, to see my doctor," she said, softening just a bit, I thought.

I asked her whether there were any symptoms she could describe other than the general run-down feeling she had mentioned. She was very positive that there were none. I asked her whether she had had any illnesses in the past, any medical history at all, and was there something specific she was being seen for in New York?

"No, I am generally very healthy. I did have a problem, but it's well under control now," she said.

"What was that?" I inquired.

"About ten years ago, my gynecologist found a cyst on one of my ovaries. As I had gone through menopause easily some years before, he recommended surgery. So I had my uterus and ovaries removed. The cyst turned out to be premalignant. Lucky we got it out in time, he told me. He also prescribed some chemotherapy, Cytoxan, which I got by vein, daily for a week. Still do, once every two or three years, when I go back to New York to see him. He's terrific. I really believe he saved me from cancer."

Yes, she confirmed, she was also being followed here, at our ob-gyn clinic, and all was fine, no complaints or unusual findings.

I was somewhat taken aback at this unorthodox treatment schedule, chemotherapy once every few years using a minimally active drug, but I said nothing, not wishing to annoy her. However, a nagging question was sitting at the back of my mind. Could this have anything to do with her current condition? Chemotherapy with Cytoxan—particularly when given alone and as a single drug so irregularly, in this fashion—surely wouldn't do much for a hidden cancer. And she seemed free of ovarian cancer, as attested to by our specialists. On the other hand, might the chemotherapy have somehow affected her immune system negatively? Could she be harboring some previously latent chronic infection, now smoldering as a very low-grade and highly localized focus? This could certainly account for the hitherto unexplained anemia and raised ESR.

One of the first things that came to mind was tuberculosis. At the time she had grown up, most people would have been exposed to the TB bacillus by adulthood. Only a minority went on to develop the full-blown overt disease. The majority overcame the initial site of infection, usually (but not only) in the lung, isolating and neutralizing it by means of an immune and local inflammatory response. The germs, however, were not always eradicated and could lie there dormant for decades, only to become reactivated coincident with some change in the person's immune system. This change could come about as a result of some other disease or drug treatments of the sort Bella had been undergoing over the years.

"Have you ever had TB?" I asked.

"No, I haven't," she answered flatly.

"Have you ever been in contact with anyone who had TB?" I asked.

"No, I have never known anyone with this illness." She was equally firm.

She was certainly old enough to have known people with TB.

"Perhaps someone in the family?" I persisted.

"No."

She was losing patience with my repetitive questions, so I decided to proceed to the physical examination.

"I would like to examine you now," I said, getting up. Her reaction was startling.

She jumped up. "No," she said. "I have had enough of examinations. I've been examined by every doctor in every one of your hospital departments, and I have had every kind of test done. Numerous needles have been jabbed into me, blood taken so many times that my arm looks like a pincushion, chest X-rays, barium meal swallows, the works. I am not being subjected to any more tests. That is all I have to say on the matter. The subject is closed."

We seemed to be back at square one—an impasse.

"Look, I only want to examine you. I promise I won't suggest you have any more tests. I cannot help you if you don't let me look at you," I said.

She considered for a moment. She looked as though she was about to refuse.

"All right, then, but no tests. You're the last doctor I intend to see. After you, I'm going to just let whatever it is take its own way. I'll live with it. I'm really good at accepting whatever fate chooses to hand out to me."

At the time I did not yet catch the underlying meaning of that last sentence.

In those days my office was the size of a matchbox. There was no place for the patient to disrobe decently, behind a screen. There was just my overflowing desk and a couch heaped with papers and X-rays. I swept the papers onto the desk, moved to the door, and asked her to undress while I left the room.

"When you are ready, please cover yourself with the sheet and I will come back into the room to examine you."

I left the room to wait outside. The temperature was rising. Patients complained, nurses were at the end of their tether. I knew I had to complete the examination and get back to the ward where I was needed.

I knocked at my door and went in. She was lying on the couch, covered to the chin by the sheet. I examined her head, neck, and chest, with Bella clutching the sheet to her waist. I then wanted to continue my examination of her abdomen and lower limbs, only to realize that she hadn't taken off her pants.

"Why haven't you fully undressed?" I asked in surprise.

"I didn't think it was necessary. None of the other doctors asked me to undress the lower part."

I couldn't believe it.

"Do you mean to say that during all these examinations you told me about earlier, no one had ever asked you to undress fully? Did no one here ever examine your belly, your groin, and your legs?" I asked disbelievingly.

"No one examined me below my chest," she insisted.

"Well, I am going to have to ask you to take off your pants, as I cannot perform a complete examination without looking at your whole body," I said.

She refused and argued with me that it simply wasn't necessary. I insisted. Again we were at an impasse.

"Is there any special reason that you do not want to take your off your slacks?" I finally asked.

"Well, I don't like people seeing my prosthesis," she said quite casually, completely unaware of the bombshell she had just delivered.

I was flabbergasted.

"What prosthesis? You never mentioned any prosthesis," I said, not letting on how shocked I was by the turn things had taken.

"Yes, well, there was no need, was there? After all, what has my artificial leg to do with anything? It happened so many years ago and has never given me any trouble, so why should I show it to the doctors and the nurses who can then gossip about me behind my back? I work here, you know. True, I am a volunteer, but I consider this my domain."

"But how did you manage to do all these tests without anyone seeing your leg?" I asked.

"Well, no one ever asked," she said simply. "They were all fixated on my test results."

This seemed so improbable to me that I was uncertain how to continue. Could she be making this up? Surely it was not possible that no one had given her a proper complete physical examination. After all, it's the first thing every student is taught in medical school. A proper examination includes the whole body, and in those days, pre- CTs and MRIs, the art of history taking and manual examination were of paramount importance. I personally believe it still is, despite technological progress and precision. She seemed quite rational and firm about what she was saying.

"All right," I said, "but now that you have told me about your prosthesis, surely you will not have any objection to my examining you properly."

Reluctantly she agreed, allowing me to complete my examination, including a thorough look and palpation of the stump below her knee, which revealed nothing new.

"Please get dressed," I said. "I would like to talk to you some more."

Once she was dressed and seated opposite me again, I asked her to tell me her story in full.

"What else do you want to know? I have already told you everything you need to know," she said crossly.

"Well, why don't you start by telling me how you came to lose your leg?" I said.

"What has that got to do with anything?" she countered.

"Just humor me," I said.

"Well, all right, if you insist, though I don't see the relevance of any of this to my present condition. I grew up in New York, a Bronx schoolgirl like all my friends, a normal childhood until I developed an infection in my shinbone when I was thirteen years old. Osteomyelitis, it's called, I now know. There were no antibiotics at the time, and the doctors tried to save my leg with repeated operations. After two horrible years, it got to an oozing stage and had to be amputated. That's all there is to the story," she said with heavy finality.

"It must have been very difficult growing up as a teenager with such a disability," I said. "How did you cope?"

"Well, you get used to everything that fate deals out to you. You make the best of it," she said dispassionately.

I now grasped the import of the sentence she had uttered at the beginning of our meeting. I realized that her apparent fatalism was only skin deep and that, in fact, the woman seated in front of me was still a hurting little girl who had had to grow up contending with a harsh world outside—minus a leg.

"What did you do when you left school?" I probed a little further.

"I went to college and qualified as a medical secretary. I stayed in New York. I felt more at home there than anywhere else. Rented a small apartment and went on my own to find a job," she said rather proudly.

"And what kind of job did you get?" I asked, thinking that it couldn't have been easy in those days to secure a position with such a disability.

"Well, after quite a few interviews, I landed a job as medical secretary in the emergency department at Bellevue Hospital. Maybe it was what I had gone through as a kid, but I really liked working with the nurses and doctors there. I often helped out with moving the patients around, taking them up for X-rays, even rushing specimens to the labs when there were urgent tests to be done. You know what a shambles the scene at Bellevue was like back then. But what I really liked most was to join the medical students on rounds, listening to them present their cases to the senior resident, watching them examining the patients. I often stayed on after my shift, tagging along with the students for hours. My leg never gave me any trouble. Maybe that's where I got started on what I've been doing here—you know, working on these medical manuscripts, which I still find so interesting."

Then a rather sad look came over her face. She sighed and fell silent. Recovering after a brief moment, she resumed her businesslike tone. "Anyway, to cut a long story short, I met my husband seven years later. He was a real Zionist, an accountant by profession. All he wanted to do was pack up and move to Israel. So that's what we did. Got married in 1954, packed our few belongings, and got on the boat to Israel."

"Do you have any children?" I asked.

"No, we could never have children. We tried, but it never worked out. The doctors gave me a million tests but said everything was OK. It was just bad luck, they said."

Again, the dispassionate note, but my ear was more attuned now to the undertones, and again I felt the hurt beneath her assumed nonchalance. I felt I needed to keep her talking.

"What does your husband do these days?" I asked by way of drawing her out a little more. So much can be learned from what the patient is telling you, as well as from the sense of what she is keeping back.

"He's no longer my husband," she said. "He left me some years ago. You see, he really wanted children, and I couldn't give him any. He found a nice, healthy American girl and went back to the States with her. He never liked it much here anyway. He has a nice, large family now, three children—two boys and a girl—and six grandchildren. He sometimes phones to ask how I am. I suppose he feels guilty. I always tell him fine and ask after his family. He raves about the grandchildren. One day they all came for a visit to Israel. He phoned, wanted to meet. I said I was busy."

All this in that same somewhat removed tone I had observed previously. It was almost as though she were talking about someone else.

"Have you ever remarried?" I asked gently.

"No," she said, "I find it easier to live my life alone."

Her sad relating of her childlessness reminded me again of TB. It was a common cause of female infertility back then, a small focus settling in the lining of the uterus, remaining dormant and inactive there but enough to interfere with conception.

Again, I approached the subject delicately. "Are you sure that no one in your family had TB?" I asked.

"I have already answered that question; my answer hasn't changed in the past half an hour that I have been in your office," she said, shaking her head as if surprised at my failing memory.

Not wishing to aggravate her again, I attempted to return to where we had left off. "Listening to your Bellevue story, I was sure you were going to tell me that you had considered going to medical school yourself."

At first, she just stared at me blankly, and then she abruptly turned her head away from me. A few minutes passed quietly with just the sound of the whirling fan above our heads emitting its creaking whistle.

"How do you know that?" she asked and then, heaving a sigh, added, "I did really want to study medicine, but it didn't work out."

Sensing that we had reached a crucial point in our discourse, I persevered. "From what you've told me about yourself then and now, it seemed obvious to me that you may have thought of becoming a doctor yourself. I would venture to speculate that you would have been a natural."

I saw the first tears in her eyes and then her quiet weeping, through which I sat in silence. Then she took a deep breath, dried her eyes with the handkerchief she'd been twisting in her hands, and faced me squarely.

"I really haven't been entirely honest with you. I didn't get to the medical school stage because I got sick. About three years after starting at Bellevue, they found a spot or two on my lung in a routine X-ray. They sure didn't mince their words. 'You've contracted lung tuberculosis,' I was told. I had never coughed up any phlegm, and I really wasn't feeling sick at all, but there were no two ways about it. Catching TB was very common in hospital personnel in those times. So I had to leave my job. They arranged for me to enter a sanatorium, up in the Adirondacks, where I would continue working as a medical secretary while I took my cure. I was given injections of streptomycin every two or three days, and another vile-tasting liquid medicine called PAS. It wasn't a bad place, you know—a bungalow village, surrounded by the woods, a lake of its own. The town nearby had a cinema and a great public library; the people were OK, those not too sick and able to socialize. Anyhow, I guess I was lucky. My X-rays mostly cleared up after six months of treatment, and after a year I was declared cured and able to leave.

"I didn't want to go back to Bellevue and didn't contact my friends there. I decided not to tell anyone about my illness. Back in the fifties, people weren't too happy to have someone around them who'd just been discharged from a TB sanatorium. Using my diploma I was able to get a job at the office of an orthopedic surgeon. Then I met my husband. We were married two years later. I never told him either. Not even when we were going through trying to have children. I guess I really buried that chapter of my life very deeply away. I have never till this moment told anyone about it."

Then she was silent, her eyes glued to the windblown eucalyptus outside my window.

I looked at Bella, and a host of thoughts flooded my mind. What inner forces had she been grappling with in persistently concealing her bad brush with TB and the impact it had had on her life? How amazing it was that if not for my instinctive attempt to keep her talking, once she had overcome her reluctance to discuss her infirmity and the life paths down which it had led her, she would have persisted in her denial.

My hunch might have been right after all.

"Look, Bella," I said, "I want to be frank with you. I think that there is a good chance that what is bothering you now is some form of reactivation of that old TB infection, a leftover from those years, some small focus somewhere in your body. Not dramatic, not enough to show up on the chest X-ray you recently had, but quite possibly enough to cause the high ESR and even the anemia. It shouldn't be too difficult to find out—"

"No way," she interrupted me forcefully. "You promised no more tests, and I really meant what I said before. No way. All I need is for someone in the hospital to find out you're thinking I have TB. This place is my entire life. My work is all I have now, and I don't intend losing it again just because some young know-it-all doctor thinks I may still have the damned bug in me somewhere."

She was very determined and getting a little more stubborn. It was now becoming clearer why she had so doggedly hidden away her true story, why she was still so adamantly averse to any further investigations. I tried to reassure her that her secret was safe with me.

"Look," I said, "no one is going to know anything about our discussion today. Even if I'm right, it has no bearing on anyone else; it's nowhere near the contagious kind of TB you remember from those years. You're not endangering anyone, and I'm under no obligation to report this."

She looked at me, contemplating, her eyes asking what I meant.

"What I propose we do is deal with this entirely the empirical way. I'd like to put you on a combination of anti-TB antibiotics. We only use pills these days, no injections or bitter-tasting syrups. The medicines don't have severe side effects, though we'll need to watch your blood tests periodically, at least initially. I figure that if all goes smoothly, we should know in six months' time whether we were right. If your ESR goes down and hemoglobin goes up, we'll say bingo and have a drink together!"

At that she smiled, the first smile she had displayed in the hour we had been talking.

"OK, Doc," she said, "you're on." She held out her hand, which I shook enthusiastically.

And that was it. I wrote out a prescription for Isoniazid and Ethambutol pills and walked her to the ward entrance.

"You know," she said in parting, "after all that, you may not find it so easy to get rid of me. But I'll tell you what. If your idea works, I'll be glad to edit your next manuscript free of charge. You'll see, it'll really come out much better than if you write it yourself."

"I'm sure you're right," I said, "and gladly accept your offer." We shook hands again, and she was off.

Needless to say, it worked. I probably wouldn't be recounting this story if it hadn't. We doctors remember, and like to recount, our successful hunch stories, not the ones that failed.

She tolerated the pills well, and within three months her ESR had fallen to normal and her anemia had cleared entirely. It was all I could do to convince her to take the full six months of treatment I thought she needed, but she finally agreed, although she fought me stubbornly all the way.

Later, we met occasionally on the hospital grounds. We would exchange greetings and a small knowing smile. She was quite a lady.

5.

HEROES DON'T CRY

The year was 1972, and I was on top of the world.

It was my second year at Moffit Hospital at the University of California Medical Center in San Francisco. Having recently finished my residency in internal medicine in Israel, I had won an international fellowship grant for training in clinical pharmacology, which enabled me to get to the United States for two years of advanced training in this field at one of the best centers in the world. I felt truly privileged to be one of the group of eight young doctors from all over the globe who'd also had the good fortune to join the training and research program run by our charismatic department chief, Dr. Ken Melmon.

It was an amazing crew to be part of and a time of endless stimulation and discovery. I was flying high, electrified both intellectually and physically. My troubled country seemed far away. Life here was normal. There was no war looming just around the corner. Vietnam was remote to a foreigner only temporarily in the United States, and anyway had by then reached the end stage of the Paris peace talks. I was entirely focused on and engrossed with this gathering of bright young people who shared my interests and enthusiasm. There were endless discussions and debates during the week, with hiking, bicycling, and lots of beer on the weekends. The decades that have flown by since have probably tinged those wonderful San Francisco years with a rosy glow, as often happens when we look back on our early days in the profession, but in my memory, and to this very day, this was a time of hitherto unfelt adventure and discovery.

In the world of academic medicine in Israel of those early years, teaching was done very much in the traditional European style. Professors wielded great authority, and young doctors were expected to listen respectfully, keep their thoughts to themselves, and certainly not question the wisdom of their elders. Here, in the environment created by Melmon, I found quite a different style of nurturing. His teaching method was Socratic, leading us to understanding by posing provocative questions and criticizing our responses very aggressively. He challenged us to think, to question any authority, and to believe that our opinions and ideas were as good as anybody else's, provided we could demonstrate that they were based on good evidence. We were encouraged to propose topics for research projects, discussions in which everyone would gleefully join to support or criticize until the idea was adopted, or more often, dropped and replaced by another.

Although we competed with each other in those debates, we were also always there to offer mutual help whenever asked in the day-to-day running of our own projects. Melmon encouraged us to attend seminars and lectures outside our own specialty program but available to us on campus, stimulating our curiosity and broadening our involvement in the main themes of scientific discourse of those times. I remember thinking that the young men of Plato's Academy in ancient Athens must have felt the same kind of exhilaration as I did. In short, life was grand.

Early one Sunday morning, I was sitting at the bay window of our rented apartment in the Sunset neighborhood, idly watching the fog roll in over Golden Gate Park, the tips of the towers of the bridge barely jutting through. I had intended to catch up with some work, but the slow motion of the fog had me mesmerized and my thoughts were drifting. My wife and sons were still asleep, and I too was nodding off, when the phone rang. I have relived that moment many times since, and although thirty years have passed, I can still feel that shrill sound ripping through my drowsy musings.

It was my old friend Ethan, phoning to say hello and tell me that he would be passing through San Francisco during the week, and could we meet. At the time there was no intimation that this was in any way a signal of distress; there was nothing dramatic about it. I have asked myself time and time again whether I could have realized that this was more than just a casual call. I have searched my memory over and over again for clues, any hint hidden in that first conversation that might have led me to suspect anything out of the ordinary. Nothing has ever surfaced.

Ethan and I had been friends forever, having grown up together as children in Jerusalem and shared many teenage escapades. The first time I laid eyes on him was through a cloud of disheveled hair, a bloody nose, and a melee of swinging arms and legs. It was 1949. I had just come to Israel from New York with my sister and parents, and this was my first day at school in Jerusalem. Although my Hebrew was fluent thanks to my father's insistent tutoring throughout my boyhood in America, some of the boys had made fun of my American accent and taunted me for my different form of dress. Boys my age had come through the War of Independence, the siege of Jerusalem, and were very much into army-style apparel, hobnailed military boots and puttees being very much the rage. I was the odd man out, neatly dressed in carefully ironed short pants and white shirt and shined lace-up shoes.

Words quickly turned into blows, and the fight was well under way when Ethan appeared on the scene. We were only ten-year-old boys, but he already had an undeniable air of authority about him, a charisma that made other boys defer to him. He came to my rescue by ending the fight, and we became firm friends. His family was well known in the city, which was then so tiny and provincial. His father, an Austrian immigrant of the 1930s, was a prominent lawyer and society man. He fell from grace several years after I met Ethan. Evidently, he had mismanaged clients' funds left in trust with him. With his father's reputation gone, along with most of his practice, Ethan, fourteen by then, oldest of four children, became the center of his doting mother's life. Working at odd jobs to augment the family income, he also became the source of authority and discipline for his younger brothers and sister.

Ethan and I were inseparable. As we grew up, we shared a love of music and listened together to his parents' collection of opera records on the cold winter nights of Jerusalem. We frequented the YMCA auditorium where the Kol Israel Symphony Orchestra held its rehearsals free, concert tickets being too expensive for us. He seemed to attract all the prettiest girls at school without making any particular effort and was always in the midst of a swirl of flirtations and early sexual encounters, which left me full of admiration tinged with envy.

Our paths diverged when we were eighteen. Ethan couldn't wait to join the army and enlisted a month after we graduated from high school. I had decided to become a doctor and went directly to medical school on a ROTC-like program and joined the army as a medical officer only seven years later, after completing my internship. While I was sweating through anatomy and physiology, Ethan excelled in the military, completing officer training school in record time. We all knew that after his compulsory thirty months, he would sign on as a regular army career officer. True to character, he did indeed stay in the military. Over the following years, we saw much less of each other, but the feelings of friendship were as strong as ever.

The Six-Day War brought us together again. As a medical officer serving in the airborne brigade, I was sent to the front about three weeks before the war began, and it was there that I met up with Ethan, now a major temporarily commanding a battalion in the same division my reserve medical outfit was attached to. During the three-week lull before the fighting erupted, we had time to catch up, play chess at night, and talk of our ambitions and dreams for the future. There was no doubt in our minds that we would come through the upcoming fighting unscathed. My plans were simple enough. After completing my residency training in internal medicine, I hoped to go to the States for a fellowship at UCSF. He was ready to leave the army and was going to be an architect or a town planner. His dream was to create a new kind of community center, possessed of "soul," as he put it, which would replace the uniform square, unimaginative buildings in the many hastily conceived new towns that dotted the country like so many discarded Lego cubes.

War solidifies and deepens bonds between men serving together, and so it was with Ethan and me. During the week of fighting, I witnessed Ethan's extraordinary courage and sangfroid. His men worshipped him and followed him into battle without hesitation. He was the kind of officer every army dreams of: intelligent, cool, rational, disciplined, a natural leader of men. He was tough but sensitive. Those who didn't know him thought he was unfeeling when he showed little emotion over the casualties, but I saw him hold his tears in check when he came to see the wounded we were treating, and recognized his agony over the dead and dying.

And then the war was over. Although it was soon to be labeled the Six-Day War, in fact it took a lot longer for me to be demobilized. Afterward we saw less and less of each other, and then Ethan was gone, off to the States to study architecture. At that time there was no e-mail, and telephone calls abroad were prohibitively expensive. Letter writing was time consuming and soon dwindled to a trickle. Finally, all that remained were a few sporadic postcards on birthdays and festive occasions. The last I heard from him was that he was marrying an American girl and settling down in Arizona, where his prospective father-in-law ran a building company.

And now this unexpected telephone call. He'd written to my parents to ask for my address and number. Not that he wanted to chat, just to let me know that he was coming to San Francisco in a few days' time and really wanted to see me.

We arranged to meet the following week. Waiting for him at a coffee place on Union Street, I saw him before he saw me. He had not changed much, straight-backed and tall, very dark with piercing brown eyes, an elongated face accentuated by a short, dark beard and a military-style crew cut. A truly striking figure of a man, he walked with a long, loose stride but gave the impression of being in a hurry. His mouth broke into a wide smile when he saw me, and we embraced; it was as if time had stood still. We quickly exchanged small talk and news of home; his parents, brothers, and sister; my family; and common friends. As I enthused over my own American experience, I couldn't help notice that there was a sense of unease between us, that his eyes stayed reserved, withdrawn. He had not mentioned his wife or children, and clearly I was expecting him to tell me about them. After a while he fell silent. I felt I would have liked to have been able to read his thoughts, sensing that he was trying to make up his mind whether to confide in me.

Finally, he resumed speaking, hesitantly and in broken phrases. "My wife and I broke up two years ago. Our divorce was nasty. Her parents and brother naturally took her side, and their constant interference precluded any kind of amicable settlement. They are a particularly vindictive family, and they blame me for ruining their daughter's life. They managed to appropriate my children and turn them against me. The situation became unbearable. There was no option. A prolonged fight in court would have harmed my two children. I had to accept separation from them and moved to Boston."

He fell silent, his jaws clenched and grinding. His misery was so bare to the eye, so at odds with his hitherto confident and strong persona, that I found it difficult to reconcile the man sitting before me with the image of the Ethan I had known in the past.

"Do you manage to see your children at all?" I asked.

"Very rarely. They don't really want to see me. They are very young, you see, and have been brainwashed into believing that I am not part of their lives anymore. When I suggest that they come to me for their summer holidays, they are always too busy. It's either camp or holidays with their grandparents. I can't really blame them."

It was clear that he had given up hope that he would ever be reunited with his children.

"Have you managed to form any new relationship since you moved away? Are you seeing anyone?" I asked, suddenly conscious of the fact that my question sounded more like a medical consultation rather than a conversation between two close friends. Ethan didn't seem to notice.

"Actually, I've found a wonderful girl, and we moved in together. I'm even thinking of getting married again," he said in a tone that belied the optimism of his words.

For a moment I sensed his unhappiness so strongly that I was at a loss for words. The Ethan I had known in childhood and in later years would have been capable of dealing with any situation. He had been through so much, first when his father was ruined and then later during the war. Of course, the present situation was different, but countless others had undergone the same losses and pain and had managed to patch up their lives. I was sure that he would come through this just as he had in the past through other difficult times. I was about to express these rather banal words of comfort when Ethan suddenly got up, saying he had a plane to catch, that he would keep in touch, and within seconds was gone.

It was only after he left that I realized that although I had babbled on and on about what I was doing, he had made no mention at all of his own work. Architecture had been the stuff of his dreams. During the war and later he had talked of nothing else, yet now he had not said a word about it throughout our talk. He had drawn me out about my medical career, and I had spent precious time enthusing about my American experience, but I had not found time or insight to ask him about his own career before his sudden departure. I also realized that he had not left a phone number where he might be reached. He had simply promised to keep in touch.

It was several months before I heard from him again. He said he hadn't been feeling well for quite some time. He'd been to see several doctors and had many tests done with no clear diagnosis made. Might they be hiding something bad from him? Could it be cancer that they weren't telling him about?

"Look, Ethan, as it happens I am going to be in Boston next week. I will be happy to see you again. We could look at your tests together and examine your options. Just give me your address and phone number."

After a moment's hesitation, Ethan agreed.

The following week I arrived at the address he had given me. It turned out to be his girlfriend's apartment in a nice residential area on the outskirts of Boston proper. I was taken aback when I first met Rita. Ethan had always been surrounded by good-looking girls, and so I suppose I had expected his present partner to conform to the pattern. The woman who greeted me with reserve at the door was a big lady, very full and rather homely. Her hair was tightly pulled back into a bun, and she was dressed casually in baggy gray trainers, which were unbecoming to her figure. She seemed to me to be older than Ethan and, at first glance, subdued in her expression.

But then she smiled, and within seconds my first impressions were forgotten. She radiated warmth and humor and welcomed me to her home as though she had known me all her life. She felt she knew me well because Ethan had often talked of me, spinning out endless stories about our Jerusalem days. I found her absolutely charming. Ethan was truly lucky to have found such a lovely person to share his life with.

He was a little thinner than when I saw him last, and somewhat apathetic. He complained of a constant lack of energy, a loss of appetite, and generally a miserable feeling of not being well. Yes, he had lost some weight, and, yes, he hadn't been sleeping so well lately. I asked to see the tests, which had been performed at a very prestigious Boston hospital. He produced a sheaf of papers. Almost everything technologically possible at the time had been done, and all the tests were negative. Nothing in the sheaf of results even hinted that something bad was lurking in his body. I then examined him thoroughly but found nothing out of the ordinary. Trying to get a better understanding of what was bothering him, I asked him about his daily routine.

"Have there been any changes at the office or in the way you spend your time after work? Do you see friends, go to the movies, read, jog?"

He smiled wryly. "I am working hard, but I manage to play squash twice a week. As for friends, I don't have many here, never did. My friends are all at home in Israel. But I have Rita; she's my best friend."

I told Ethan that I saw no basis whatsoever for his belief that he had some sort of cancer. I thought that given the negative result of the thorough medical workup he'd had and the nature of his symptoms, it was very likely that he was suffering from a mild form of depression. I suggested he seek help from a psychiatrist, who would be better equipped than I to advise and treat him.

Ethan reacted very badly to my suggestion. He had no need of psychiatrists, thank you very much. He was fine mentally, not crazy. It was just that whatever it was hiding inside him had not yet been identified by the doctors. He was sure that it was there, and with time I would realize that he was right about his self-diagnosis.

I remonstrated with him. "Ethan, depression is an illness just like any other. There is no distinction between body and mind. Brain cells and chemicals can malfunction biologically just like any other organ. Surely you understand that going to a psychiatrist doesn't mean you're crazy. There are new, effective drugs to help alleviate depression."

He would not accept anything I said. Antidepressant drugs had side effects, he said. He had heard of people who had become impotent as a result of taking those drugs. And anyway, he was not depressed. He turned to Rita, stroking her hair gently. "Tell him that there is nothing wrong with me up here," he said, pointing to his head. "Whatever it is, it's somewhere inside me, below this line." He now placed his hand horizontally, at the level of his Adam's apple, with a rueful glance at Rita.

She confirmed that there had been no change in his daily routine, other than his preoccupation with the possibility that he was much sicker than the doctors were telling him.

Ethan was getting upset, so I decided to back off for a while to let him cool down and reconsider the course of action I had suggested. I was going back to San Francisco that evening but would be back in Boston a fortnight later. We agreed to meet again then.

On the way out, Rita accompanied me to the bus stop. I asked her again whether there had been any change she didn't want to mention in his presence. No, she said, repeating what she had already told me.

"How is his work going?" I asked. "Is he satisfied with the way his career is progressing? Are there any problems at the office?"

Quite to the contrary, she said and explained that he now was heading the team designing a big construction complex for a multinational company and was very excited about the task. He had been chosen for the project over many of his competitors and was very proud of it. He had the plans spread out all over the house and was constantly pointing out to her the groundbreaking ideas in his design.

I left her with my thoughts. I told her I still thought that Ethan was indeed suffering from mild depression brought on by the divorce and separation from his children. Perhaps it was also being exacerbated by pressure at work, burdened as he was by the responsibility for the new project he was so deeply involved in. Would she please keep in touch and let me know how things were going? I asked. I hoped to see them again two weeks hence and try once more to persuade him to see a psychiatrist if he wasn't improved by then.

Two days later, back in San Francisco, I phoned Ethan to ask how he was.

"Much better," he said. He sounded almost gay. "Rita and I are considering going away on holiday when I finish working on the building plans. It should be quite soon. She wants to go to Hawaii. Have you ever been there?"

I said I had indeed and could wholeheartedly recommend a vacation there. I was very pleased that they were planning a holiday and felt relieved that his mood had so improved.

The phone rang again at noon the next day. It was Rita, her voice dull, mechanical. Ethan was dead. He'd killed himself, jumped off the roof of their building that very morning.

I was numb with shock and disbelief. It was not possible that Ethan had committed suicide. I had seen him at war, under the most terrible duress. I had been with him when he assumed responsibility for other men's lives, had shared his anguish when some of his men were killed. I had watched him fight off the torment of guilt over their deaths and seen him proceed to the next battle cool and calm as always. Surely this was not the kind of man who would put an end to his own life. He had assured me only the other day that he was doing better.

Disbelief gave way to grief. I would never see Ethan again. Although we had drifted apart in those last years, he had always been a significant part of my life. Friendships formed in childhood are not easily erased. Now everything we had shared would be relegated to memory, fading with time, leaving a deep void. Finally, guilt set in. What signal had I missed? How could I have not sensed the severity of his depression? Could I have detected any hints of suicidal intent? Could I have prevented Ethan from taking this terrible final step?

I went to Boston for the funeral. His ex-wife and children were there, as well as his parents, brothers, and sister from Jerusalem. Rita, still in shock, cried all the time. The service was mercifully short, and the grave was quickly covered.

Back in Rita's apartment, it became apparent that nobody was aware of Ethan's depression. His parents knew nothing of it, nor did his brothers and sister. They showed me his letters, which they had brought with them from Israel. They were cheerful, even humorous, and gave no hint of anything wrong, even those written in recent weeks. He was planning a visit home and asking the family whether there was anything he could bring them from the States. He described his new architectural project and was obviously very excited and happy about it. There were some references to Rita, leading the family to surmise that he was serious about her. Ethan's mother collapsed in tears, saying that she had imagined herself coming to the States for his wedding, never dreaming that she would finally meet Rita at his funeral.

Ethan's ex-wife, a cool, well-groomed brunette, also had no knowledge of any depression. True, she had not seen much of Ethan since the divorce, but he communicated with the children every now and again. She had not had any intimation of anything wrong. Yes, the divorce had ended badly; Ethan was a difficult man. The cultural chasm between Phoenix and Jerusalem might have been just too wide to bridge. But in the last few months, she had actually talked to Ethan on the phone about the children and even acceded to his wish to take them to Boston during the summer holidays. Communication between them had been reestablished, and it seemed to her that they were on the way to a more amicable relationship.

It was getting late, and everyone left. Rita and I remained alone. I made us some tea; she was so forlorn, seemingly at the end of her tether.

"I know it's difficult to believe that I knew nothing about his depression," she said, "but I didn't. I could feel his mother thinking, 'Why didn't she do anything to stop him? Why didn't she call us and tell us he was troubled?' You must believe me; I truly thought he was happy with me and that the only thing troubling him was the thought that the doctors had misdiagnosed his illness. He made me promise not to tell his parents about his cancer fears. He said that would worry them needlessly. I agreed not to tell them on condition that he went to see you in California to hear your opinion. He came back from your reunion without having told you about it.

"After your visit with us here, he began to tone down his cancer worries, but he couldn't accept the label of depression nor bear the idea of psychiatric treatment, especially coming from you, his friend. You asked me at the time whether there was any change in his pattern of behavior, and I said no. But after his suicide, it came to me that there was one thing that had certainly changed after he came back from meeting you in San Francisco. He stopped watching the news broadcasts on television. Ethan had always been obsessive about watching the news, and he never missed the evening program, to see if anything bad had happened back home."

Rita continued, "I always kidded him about it, and he used to say that it was a habit acquired in Israel, where everyone listens to the news several times a day. Anyhow, after he came back from seeing you the first time, he suddenly stopped, even walking out of the room when I turned the TV on. After your visit with us here, he also stopped reading the morning paper. Could this have been a weird reaction to what you told him? I should have told you about it when you asked, but it seemed so trivial at the time that I didn't think it worth mentioning. Now I could shoot myself for not telling you. Perhaps it would have made a difference."

This monologue seemed to have sapped her strength, and within minutes she fell asleep on the sofa. I let myself out quietly and went to my hotel. I was exhausted but couldn't sleep. I tossed and turned and finally gave up on sleep altogether to wait for morning.

I thought about Rita. Surely she must have noticed other changes in Ethan's behavior besides the one she had told me about. Was it possible that in keeping with his pattern of denial, she too had allowed herself to be led into believing there was nothing seriously wrong? She must have realized that had she told me about those changes, I possibly would have recognized his depression as more severe and perhaps done more to convince or even force him to seek psychiatric help. Why then didn't she confide in me?

My thoughts then drifted to my last meeting with Ethan. Had I been wrong to suggest that his problem was mental and not physical? Given his obvious fear of psychiatric treatment, which labeled him in his own eyes as crazy, would it have been better to let him go on believing that he had cancer? Had I been grossly wrong in trying to disabuse him of this belief? Could I have had more insight, or spent more time with him, to help him become reconciled to the thought that the right course of action was to arrange for professional treatment by a psychiatrist?

Morning finally came and I could get outdoors for my run, hoping the exercise would help deaden the feelings of overwhelming guilt and sorrow that were tearing me up. The air was cold and the wind biting, clearing my head. As I ran past some newly built apartment blocks, it suddenly came to me that I had not seen Ethan's actual building project, only the plans Rita had shown me. Perhaps I could get the address from Rita and go over to take a look, possibly getting a better perspective of Ethan's frame of mind through seeing his work. After breakfast I called Rita. She sounded better than the night before and gave me the addresses of Ethan's office and the building site.

I went over to the office first, thinking that perhaps someone working with Ethan might be able to explain the project to me. It then occurred to me that it was strange that no one from his office had come to the funeral. I had not thought of it before because of the shock, which we were all experiencing, but now it suddenly loomed large in my mind. I took a cab to the address that Rita had given me. It was a modern office block with only one architectural firm listed in the lobby. I took the elevator up to the twenty-fifth floor and asked the receptionist if I might speak to someone who had worked with Ethan.

She had never heard of him. She was new, she said, but she led me to Ed Wise, a senior partner in the firm. Ed was a middle-aged, rather unprepossessing man with pale blue eyes and thin, sandy hair. He was casually dressed in a roll-necked sweater and jeans and was at work at a drawing board. I presented myself, apologizing for barging in without making an appointment, explained the situation, and asked about Ethan and the project. Ed was visibly shocked. He did not know of Ethan's death. Yes, he said, Ethan had worked on the project, but he had left a long time ago.

Two years earlier, Ed told me, Ethan had been employed by the firm to assist on some relatively unimportant projects. The firm then won the contract for the new multinational building project. Everyone was ecstatic and Ethan especially so.

"He told everyone that his dream had finally come true," said Ed. "You see, it was everything he had always worked for. He hoped that now, finally, he'd be the one to design this project, the one he'd always dreamed of."

As Ed talked, a scene suddenly flashed through my mind. I remembered Ethan in his army uniform sitting on the ground of the Sinai desert and dreamily telling me about the buildings possessed of a soul that he would one day design.

"Ethan immediately began working feverishly on the building designs," Ed continued. "He dedicated every waking moment to his drafting and drove everyone in the firm berserk with his obsessive need to talk about his ideas, incessantly pestering everyone for attention. Finally, his proposal was ready. Others had also prepared their designs, and we had agreed from the beginning that everyone would pool their ideas to create the very best possible plan. At the partners' meeting, Ethan presented his design, his "baby," as he called it. It was unanimously rejected. We retained some small parts, but the rest was thrown overboard."

"Why?" I asked. "What was wrong with it?"

"The design was brilliant," said Ed, "but totally impractical in terms of the financial resources allocated to it. It would have cost at least double the sum we had at our disposal. The investors would have rejected it out of hand and would have probably fired us had we dared to present it to them."

"How did Ethan take the rejection?" I asked.

"Well, he seemed unable to accept the verdict," said Ed rather sadly, repeatedly drawing his hand through his thin hair. "He raved and ranted and tried to convince the partners that they were making a grave mistake, but they were not persuaded. His design was dumped. Ethan resigned from the firm that day, and we have not seen him since."

"What about the building complex itself?" I asked.

Ed took me to the window and pointed out a giant building site several blocks away, with workers swarming over the scaffoldings.

"There it is," he said.

I looked at it with incomprehension. Was this what Ethan's death was about? This ugly block of steel, glass, and concrete?

I remembered the numerous plans spread all over the house that Rita had said he was working on. I realized that he must have been "going to work" every morning for about a year after he left the firm. Where would he have gone? Why did he feel unable to tell Rita about his failure? Was he afraid of losing her respect or of the possibility of her leaving him? How lonely he must have been. And why could he not confide in me, his oldest friend?

Would Ethan still be alive if he had been allowed to design the building? I doubted it. But perhaps, I thought, it wasn't the rejection of the plans—the failure itself—that had gotten to Ethan so badly. Perhaps it was the loss of control. Here was a man whose whole life was about control, both of his own destiny and that of others. A hard man, unrelenting, determined to pursue his own way. A leader. And above all, always the hero. On the day of his suicide, Ethan carefully shaved, dressed neatly, ate breakfast with Rita, and then quietly went up to the roof. In making the preparation to jump, and then in the act itself, Ethan was somehow reclaiming control over his life.

I went back to San Francisco and visited the library to find Karl Menninger's *Man Against Himself*, which I had first read years before. The book may seem outdated today in light of our knowledge of genetics and neurobiology, but the main theory underpinning Menninger's work seems as true today as it was then. It was his contention that people who commit suicide are inherently self-destructive. Tracing their lives back to childhood, one will generally find a trail of self-damaging behavior reflected in the decisions they made at every significant crossroad they encountered.

Ethan's life too had been dogged persistently by a streak of recklessness and wrong choices made at each intersection. Memories came flooding back from childhood, from adolescence, from youth. There was the time Ethan and I played truant from school to go to the beach in Tel Aviv. It was deserted and black flags were up, indicating dangerous currents. Ethan and I were both good swimmers, but we had trained in the YMCA indoor pool in Jerusalem and had only rarely been to the beach. Ethan plunged right in, calling for me to follow. I hesitated but in the end followed him, as always. Within minutes we were caught in the swirling currents, and I still recall the suffocating fear and helplessness that I felt during those long moments before we were pulled out by an extremely angry lifeguard.

And then there was the time he dared me to venture out of the confines of our Jerusalem neighborhood and into the hills, beyond the Monastery of the Cross, through deserted rocky pathways to the ruins of Malcha, an abandoned and ruined Arab village. These were the days of marauders infiltrating the Judean hills, and this kind of wandering was strictly forbidden to us boys. Our parents were seriously worried and meted out severe punishments when we returned from our adventure.

As we grew up, there were several other episodes, some more hazardous, others less. I recalled the time when as young men we took our current girlfriends for an overnight hike to Masada, arriving at the base of the mountain toward evening. This was long before the time of the cable car and the conveniently well-marked paths up the mountain. In those days there was just one rough, unmarked trail leading to the top. Young people would camp at the base and commence their climb before dawn to watch the sunrise over the Dead Sea from the top.

We intended to do the same, but at two o'clock in the morning, Ethan woke us up and suggested we start the climb right then, in pitch-black darkness. It was a measure of his qualities of leadership that both the girls and I embarked on this extremely foolhardy expedition. We made it to the top, but not before one of the girls had fallen to a ledge below and had to be precariously pulled up, more frightened than badly bruised. Ethan set about persuading her that she was taking part in a great adventure and that life would be dull and colorless without risks and dangers. Within minutes he had her convinced and smiling despite her scratches, which looked pretty painful. There were many other such "adventures" in Ethan's life, some of which I participated in, others that he gleefully related to me.

I wondered about his failed marriage. I had not managed to talk much to his ex-wife during the funeral. The atmosphere had been too emotionally charged, with his parents shocked and uncomprehending, Rita crying ceaselessly, his ex-wife stony-faced, holding her children by the hand, the children themselves bewildered, and myself reeling with the trauma and self-blame. The situation was definitely not conducive to a more profound conversation with his ex-wife. But now back in San Francisco, I thought I would like to talk to her again to find out more about Ethan's state of mind before the divorce.

I realized I did not even know her name. I looked up Ethan's family name in the telephone directory in Phoenix, Arizona, hoping that she may have kept the name because of the children. I found it immediately. She had indeed kept it. I phoned, thinking that she might not be willing to talk to me and quite prepared to apologize and retreat. She was cool but cooperative, her tone of voice emotionless, almost as though she were talking about someone else. Perhaps she was holding her emotions in check, but I didn't think so.

The marriage had started off well. Ethan loved the desert landscape of Arizona and its climate, which reminded him of Israel. He was just out of architecture school and had great ambitions to create truly innovative designs. He started to work for her father, a building contractor, and at first things went well. The children were born, and all seemed set for success and happiness. Then his architectural plans became more ambitious and more expensive to build. Her father's firm could not afford the extravagance, and Ethan was asked to modify his designs to comply with the budget constraints. But he would not back down. Other architects were engaged to propose more realistic plans, and Ethan's work was finally rejected in their favor. He became embittered. Quarrels with her father ensued and finally spilled over to sour their marital relationship. He blamed her for not backing him up, for taking her father's side. Finally, she couldn't take it anymore and sued for divorce and custody of the children.

I thanked her for her openness and willingness to talk to me and wished her well.

That was as far back as I could go. Everyday life took over, and I went back to my own family and work. Soon Ethan receded into the background and finally into the recesses of memory. But I never quite managed to put the whole story out of my mind. For some years I was obsessed with the thought that if it had not been for Rita's lack of perception (or at times when my anger got the better of me, her passiveness or even stupidity), I might have saved him.

It was only now, more than thirty years later, as I was writing this story, that I finally realized that I had been blaming her all these years because I had never been able to admit to myself that I had made a terrible mistake in not recognizing the severity of Ethan's depression. I was young at the time and sure of myself. Humility comes only with age and experience. I didn't realize then that even without the telltale marks of major changes in behavior patterns, every depression is to be taken very seriously, and especially when accompanied by morbid thoughts of death such as Ethan's cancer preoccupation.

I also know today that I should have examined Ethan's past modes of behavior more closely, especially as our years of friendship afforded me a unique opportunity to do so. Had I done this, I probably would have detected signs of self-destructiveness much earlier on. I have often asked myself why it was I failed to pursue the subject of Ethan's professional life both on the first occasion of our meeting in San Francisco and then again at his home in Boston. It should have been natural for me to inquire after his career; it was insensitive on my part not to have done so. Was it possible that I had somehow sensed failure in the air and that I was reluctant to find out that my childhood hero had feet of clay? Was I perhaps uncomfortable with the contrast between my own happiness and sense of fulfillment at the time and Ethan's dejection? Could this have contributed to my mistake in judgment?

A psychiatrist friend to whom I recounted this story said, "Having misdiagnosed the severity of a depression once, you will never do it again. The alarm bells will sound loud and clear. It is something many psychiatrists learn the hard way."

I no longer blame Rita. I have also been able to accept my own role in Ethan's death. All that is left is a great sorrow for the fine life that might have been, but never was fulfilled.

6.

IN TANDEM

They walked into my office late one September afternoon soon after I had opened my consulting practice. Jonathan and Dana—an exceptionally handsome couple in their early forties, both of them tall, slim, blue-eyed, and very fair. In fact, they looked so much alike they could have been taken for brother and sister had they not made the appointment as Mr. and Mrs. Storr. As they settled into their seats, I noticed they even had a similar way of crossing their legs and placing their hands in their laps. From the outset I was struck by their close rapport, by how very much they were in tune with each other.

I asked how I could be of help. They both started speaking at once, but, with a quick glance at Jonathan, Dana took over. Since coming down with the flu about two months earlier, she said, Jonathan hadn't really recovered. He seemed to be unable to regain his strength and resume his usual hectic schedule. He still had a low-grade fever and felt constantly tired and under the weather, with no sign of improvement. Could I help them find out what the problem was?

Intrigued, I proceeded to inquire about Jonathan's medical history before examining him. The information gleaned in this way is almost always richly rewarding, and in those days, the 1970s, we had much more time to spend with our patients. Managed care wasn't about counting our minutes, nor were we so focused on the computer screen as we are today, and we could actually look at the patient as we spoke.

I began by asking what their family physician had thought and recommended. To my surprise, Dana said they did not have one. At this point Jonathan took over the reporting. This present ailment was a completely new experience to him, he said. He'd never been ill, never needed to consult a doctor, never been hospitalized for any reason.

"Not even for tonsils, appendicitis, or a broken leg?" I asked.

No, he had always been perfectly healthy, he assured me, citing the standard Israeli measure of physical fitness: the army service. As a soldier doing his national service, he was in the infantry for three grueling years, during which he had had no health problems. Later, as an officer in the reserves, he had fought in the Sinai during the Six-Day War and survived without a scratch. Dana nodded. During their ten years of marriage, she avowed, she had never seen him ill, which was why she was worried now.

We continued our talk. It turned out they were your typical high-powered couple. Jonathan was head of a successful software company he had founded six years earlier, after a promising but financially unrewarding academic career in mathematics and computer sciences. Dana was a partner in a top Tel Aviv law firm and held a PhD in international law. They were childless by choice, they explained; their careers left no time for raising a family, and besides, this country was too dangerous to raise children in. They liked to spend their vacations rock climbing. In fact, it was their favorite sport, and in two weeks' time they were planning to go on a ten-day vacation climbing in the

Dolomites. Conditions at this time of year were optimal, and arrangements to take the time off work were made months in advance. Could they proceed as planned?

I examined Jonathan. He did indeed have a low-grade fever, and he looked pale. As I examined his abdomen, I found something more worrying. His spleen was very much enlarged and firm in texture to my probing fingers. This was not something to be expected in a patient who insisted he had no record of illness until two months earlier. Spleens do not usually become so enlarged without some kind of warning sign or accompanying symptoms over a more extended period.

It seemed unlikely that the size and texture of Jonathan's spleen could be explained simply as a lingering effect of some earlier viral infection such as mononucleosis, but to rule out those options I sent him off for a panel of blood tests and a chest X-ray. The X-ray was clear, and the blood test results were all normal, other than a mild degree of anemia, and they did not they indicate mononucleosis. Nevertheless, when Jonathan returned a few days later, he wasn't feeling any better. His temperature was practically normal, he reported, but it was still 37.8 °C when I took it.

I now asked him to go to the hospital for further diagnostic work-up. At the time, there weren't as many diagnostic tests and technologies available in an ambulatory setting as there are today. We had no computerized tomography (CT scanners), and access to diagnostic ultrasound was limited. I also wanted blood cultures taken each time his temperature went up, to rule out a bacterial bloodstream infection. This could be done conveniently only in the hospital. Jonathan protested. There was too much to be done at the office, and this would surely blow over in a few days. Couldn't I just try some antibiotics or whatever? After all, the tests were OK, weren't they? I tried to sway him, but he was adamant. He would wait.

A week later Dana called. Jonathan was no better; could they check into the hospital the next morning? In the days that followed, she never left his side. Although he was only undergoing some tests and suffered no pain or discomfort, she refused to go home and spent the nights in a chair in his room. Only once a day did she leave his bedside, to change her clothes and bring him his favorite food. Not many friends came to visit. It occurred to me that the two of them were so immersed in their shared private world that they perhaps had no need for friends. One or two colleagues from Jonathan's firm dropped in, but this was still far removed from the norm in Israeli hospitals, where families and friends tend to overrun the wards, often squatting there for the duration. Dana's parents lived in the United States; Jonathan's were both dead. Neither she nor he had brothers or sisters, and they did not seem to have any other relations.

On ward rounds, I checked to see if I had missed anything the first time I saw Jonathan. I went over the notes made by the medical student assigned to record his history and compared them with the resident physician's report. There was nothing new there. Jonathan gave him, almost verbatim, the same account he had given me: there was nothing to report; his health had always been excellent. The repeated physicals had revealed no new findings, and the first routine tests were all negative, as were the blood cultures and serological tests for specific infections. Radioactive isotope uptake scans showed a greatly oversized spleen and slightly enlarged liver, but indicated nothing to clarify the ongoing process in their tissues.

In discussing the possible causes of Jonathan's condition, the staff's foremost concern was that he might have Hodgkin's disease or some other type of lymphoma (cancer of the lymph glands). We did a lymphangiogram, a radiological procedure in the pre-CT era that involved injecting a dye opaque to X-rays into the skin of the foot. Serial X-rays followed the progress of the dye up the lymph vessels of the lower limbs into the glands of the groin, pelvis, and abdomen, looking for signs indicating malignancy. The results were inconclusive; there was nothing definitive on the films.

To establish a definite diagnosis of lymphoma that would allow us to plan treatment, we needed a pathologist's examination of the spleen, as well as accurate structural details of the internal organs. Today, CT and MRI—modern imaging technologies with ultrasound—easily provide the required information. At the time, however, the best available medical procedures were exploratory surgery to examine the abdominal cavity and internal organs, and splenectomy, removal of the enlarged spleen. At this point we began considering both options. The latter would also have preempted the grave danger people in Jonathan's condition were constantly faced with: any accidental trauma to the left lower ribs or upper abdomen could rupture the swollen spleen and cause life-threatening bleeding into the abdominal cavity. Nevertheless, a decision on such major intervention was not to be taken lightly.

I found myself starting to feel uneasy about how things were unfolding. I slept badly at night, always a sure sign that something about a patient was worrying me. A vague thought, a shapeless memory, tugged at the edge of my consciousness but stubbornly eluded me. I became frustrated and, as my wife put it, very crotchety. Then early one morning, after tossing and turning for hours, I sat bolt upright in bed, having suddenly realized what had been bothering me.

The first time Jonathan came to see me, I noticed a patch of light brown discoloration on the skin of his back, which I took for a change in pigmentation caused by overexposure to the sun. Such changes are not uncommon in our Mediterranean climate; I myself have them and find it necessary to cover my face and arms when exposed to the sun. I therefore did not give the matter a second thought. In fact, I did not even recall noticing the patch until that sleepless night, when its memory suddenly resurfaced. It then took on a whole new significance.

Back in my student days, when doing my rotation in dermatology, our professor had presented to us a case of Gaucher's disease, a rare condition first described at the end of the nineteenth century by the French physician for whom it is named. Gaucher's is found mostly in Jews of east European ancestry. The cause is a mutated gene, leading to impaired disposal of breakdown substances produced in body tissues by the normal cycle of cell death and renewal.

All human cells are bounded by membranes built of large lipid (fatty substances) and protein molecules. In the normal sequence, membranes of dying cells are broken down and the lipids digested by a particular enzyme within scavenger cells, special cells found in the liver, spleen, and bone marrow. The Gaucher mutations give rise to a defective, inactive form of the enzyme. As a result, the lipids cannot be digested. Instead, they remain in the diseased scavenger cells, now known as Gaucher's cells. Over time these lipid-filled, foamy cells grow in size and number, riddling the bone marrow and leading to the enlargement of the spleen and liver.

As the disease progresses, the enlarged spleen entraps and destroys blood cells, while in the bone marrow, blood cell production is impaired by the Gaucher cells. The result may be anemia, bleeding, and impaired ability to fight off bacterial infections. The bones are also weakened structurally, and patients may suffer bone pain and even fractures. The swollen spleen is particularly prone to rupture after even minimal trauma, followed by life-threatening abdominal bleeding. Any or all of these complications may occur in the course of a Gaucher patient's lifetime. Nowadays the disease can be kept at bay thanks to a bioengineered version of the enzyme, which, given regularly, does away with all symptoms. In those years, however, it was untreatable; the natural course of its most severe form was inexorably downhill, ending almost invariably with the patient's death.

And now, at four in the morning, it suddenly came back to me: one of the earliest symptoms of Gaucher's may be the unexpected changes in skin pigmentation known as café-au-lait patches—just like the discoloration I had seen on Jonathan's back.

I had not previously considered Gaucher's a possible cause of Jonathan's enlarged spleen. His symptoms and their sudden appearance suggested Hodgkin's or some other lymphoma. While Gaucher's does sometimes appear suddenly late in adult life, it more commonly surfaces somewhere in the first three decades. Moreover, even in cases that are diagnosed only beyond that age, the patient usually suffers some form of ill health that is often only attributed to Gaucher's with hindsight, once the more distinctive symptoms have crystallized. Since Jonathan was in his early forties and perfectly healthy until the onset of his symptoms a few months back, I'd focused all my attention on the grim possibility of lymphoma. And yet Gaucher's was evidently stirring at the back of my mind.

Wide awake now, I got up and began rereading my material on Gaucher's. At first I found no mention of the coffee-colored patches, but a more intensive search produced the notes I was looking for. Things fell into place.

It could very well be, I mused, that Jonathan was indeed suffering from the disease. Perhaps he had experienced some minor symptoms over the years, which both he and Dana had disregarded. That would account for their firm belief in his perfect health. And if indeed we were dealing with Gaucher's, abdominal surgery and removal of the spleen would not only be completely superfluous but could actually aggravate the condition. In Gaucher's the spleen serves as storage space for some of the excess lipids; without it, they would overload the liver and bone marrow even more quickly and cause more damage.

The next step, I thus decided, should be a sternal puncture and bone marrow aspiration. This was a particularly unpleasant procedure for the patient, involving the insertion of a large-bore hypodermic needle into the breastbone and application of suction through a syringe to draw out the bone marrow tissue. Microscopic examination of the cellular material would identify the telltale foamy Gaucher cells and confirm my hunch.

That morning at the hospital, I went at once to Jonathan's room to share my thoughts about his symptoms and the required course of action, and to prepare him for the procedure. Dana was there as usual—beautiful, cool, smartly dressed. Jonathan sat up in bed, freshly shaven, wearing crisp pajamas, his blond hair still wet from the shower. Almost too stereotypical to be true, I thought, Barbie and Ken. None of their obviously intense feelings for each other showed in their faces. Their joint response to my words was controlled, almost mechanical, as if maintaining the perfect, cool image were of utmost importance.

Shaking off these thoughts, I turned to the job at hand and asked the two to describe to me any kind of minor symptom Jonathan had ever had. Anything, I said, such as a rash, repeated colds, a low-grade fever, headaches, sore throat, stomachaches, and diarrhea. No, nothing at all, they replied, Jonathan had always been perfectly healthy. I then began to explain what we were looking for and why I was suggesting the biopsy. I asked them whether they had ever heard of Gaucher's disease. Both had not. They wanted to know all the details and asked for as much information as possible. I explained the purpose of the biopsy and described the procedure step-by-step. As I expected, they asked many questions, all of which were pertinent.

Later that day Jonathan, cheerful and talkative as ever, was prepared for the sternal puncture: laid on his back, his chest bared, and the breastbone area swabbed with iodine and draped with sterile surgical napkins. I first infiltrated the skin with a local anesthetic injection.

Then, just as I was leaning over him with the aspiration needle at the ready, about to drill it into his breastbone, he casually remarked, "Oh, I remember this. I've been through all this before."

Utterly stunned, I stopped in mid motion. The whole room fell silent. Everyone present knew of Jonathan's exceptionally clean medical record. I put down the syringe.

"What do you mean you remember this procedure?" I demanded. "You've been telling us for days that you'd never seen the inside of a hospital, never been ill in your life." It briefly crossed my mind he might be joking with me, perhaps to allay the fear brought on by the sight of the rather large needle I was brandishing over his bare chest. "Where did you have this procedure done?"

"At Meir Hospital," he answered without a trace of embarrassment.

"Why did you hide this fact from me?"

"I didn't hide anything. It was such a long time ago, I simply forgot."

"How long ago?" I could barely contain my anger. All that time I had wasted grappling with the case, all those nights of fitful sleep spent worrying that I was getting it wrong—and here was Jonathan telling me perfectly calmly that he had been through all this before.

"I can't remember; it must have been years and years ago. Ask Dana, she might remember," he said. "But why are you so upset, Doctor?"

I got hold of myself and ignored the question. Resuming my professional cool, I said, "That is a good idea; I think I *will* ask Dana. Meanwhile, the nurse will take you back to your room."

"But, Doctor," he asked, "aren't you going to continue with the biopsy?"

I explained it might no longer be necessary and that before proceeding with any further tests we would reassess his case in light of the new information he had given us.

Dana was sitting outside on a bench, pale and concerned. "Is it over? Is Jonathan all right?"

I reassured her that Jonathan was fine and asked her to come into my office. There I told her what had transpired and asked if she remembered when Jonathan had had his previous bone marrow aspiration.

"Oh, that!" She heaved a sigh of relief that I wasn't about to give her some bad news. "I remember now. It was about ten years ago. Jonathan wasn't feeling well, and the doctor thought he should do some tests at the hospital. But they didn't find anything wrong with him."

Again, I found my temper mounting. "Why didn't you tell me about all this when I asked you whether Jonathan had ever been hospitalized? Surely you couldn't have forgotten such an experience?" I was almost shouting at her.

"Well, it wasn't really much of an experience," she responded coolly. "After all, the doctors didn't find anything wrong with Jonathan, and it didn't affect our lives in any way. So we simply forgot all about it. Why all this fuss?"

She was clearly upset by my questioning, and, treading more carefully now, I asked about the purpose of the biopsy all those years ago.

"Oh, I don't know. I think they said something about the bone marrow, but as I told you, it came to nothing. They found nothing wrong and said we could just get on with our lives and forget all about it. So we did."

I asked her whether the doctors had ever mentioned Gaucher's disease at the time. No, she said very firmly, they had not.

She was growing increasingly anxious, so I left things at that and calmed her down. We would keep Jonathan in the hospital just a little while longer, I told her, while we contacted the other hospital to obtain some information we needed.

After our talk she hurried off to Jonathan's room. When I looked in on them a little later, they were watching TV, composed and relaxed, completely oblivious, it seemed to me, to the shock my staff and I had experienced. Jonathan wanted to know how soon he could get back to work, as there were some important matters he had to deal with, and Dana asked if they could go on their planned rock-climbing holiday. I told them I would answer their questions as soon as I received information from the doctors who had treated him ten years ago. Neither Jonathan nor Dana could tell me their names, or even in which ward Jonathan had the procedure.

I began phoning the Meir internal medicine wards and was answered almost immediately by an old acquaintance, Dr. Aaron Samuel. He and I had been to medical school together and had been in touch with each other on and off for many years. As it happened, Dr. Samuel was head of the ward where Jonathan had been hospitalized, and he was very happy to help. I asked him whether he remembered Jonathan's case from ten years ago.

"You mean the Gaucher's case?" he said. "It wasn't ten years ago; it was only four—just before the Yom Kippur War.

Yes, he remembered the patient quite clearly, a very impressive young man with a big spleen. He had performed a bone marrow aspiration and diagnosed Gaucher's. As a matter of fact, he still had the microscopy slides and would gladly send them to me in the morning.

I asked Dr. Samuel if he had fully informed the couple of the results and explained to them the significance of the disease. He was slightly annoyed. Did I seriously think he would release a patient with Gaucher's from the hospital without fully informing him of the nature of his illness? Both the patient and his wife were such highly intelligent adults, so well equipped to deal with the information. He had spent a long time with them, explaining everything and answering all their questions. He talked to them at length about the potential implications of having children. And he especially emphasized the dangers of sustaining injury and counseled against any form of hazardous sport.

Dr. Samuel was as good as his word, and when I came to the hospital the next morning, I found the slides on my desk. They left absolutely no doubt: Jonathan had indeed been correctly diagnosed with Gaucher's disease four years earlier.

I asked Jonathan and Dana into my office and related to them my conversation with Dr. Samuel. By now I knew full well that there was no sense in remonstrating with them. I put it in the most straightforward fashion I could.

"We all know now that you were already diagnosed with Gaucher's four years ago. I can only repeat what Dr. Samuel told you then. There is nothing we can do for you by way of cure, but it is very important that you refrain from any activity that might result in a fall or injury of any kind, as we could not remove the spleen without endangering you. Skiing, rock climbing, any extreme sport must be ruled out for life."

They both reacted as if it were all news to them and made no effort to explain their complete silence hitherto. Once again, they took my words stoically. Not a tear was shed. No expression of anxiety or sadness marred their placid countenances. They asked their customary incisive questions and listened carefully to my replies. Their reaction no longer surprised me. I asked Jonathan to come back in three months for a routine checkup, and he promised to do so. They thanked me profusely and left hand in hand. I was quite certain they would not return.

In the months that followed, I could not get Jonathan and Dana out of my head. Even as a young physician, I was already familiar with the wide range of defense mechanisms evident in patients confronted by harsh reality. But I had never before encountered such a mechanism as this overwhelming denial, not only of the patient's but of his wife's as well. Could it be that they were so close to each other that they unconsciously threw the same veil over reality?

So troubling were these questions that I decided to take them up with Dr. Samuel. He was equally baffled and intrigued, and we decided to get together to discuss the case.

A few weeks later, we sat at his office exploring possible explanations. Perhaps it was something in their background, I said. Dr. Samuel vaguely remembered that Hedda, the head nurse in his ward at the time, had told him that Jonathan and Dana had been her neighbors for a couple of years. Perhaps she could provide some insights that would help unravel the enigma.

Nurse Hedda was now retired, but we obtained her address from the hospital records, and I had a long chat with her. Yes, she said, she remembered the couple. In fact, she knew them quite well when they were living nearby. I learned that when Jonathan was only twelve, his mother died of cancer. Then, when he was in his twenties, his father too fell ill with cancer, and Jonathan had spent over a year at the hospital, coming in every single day to see his father, and was beside himself with grief as he watched him slowly dying in great pain. Soon after his father's death, he met and married Dana.

"And what did you know about her?" I asked Hedda. Quite a lot, it turned out. In their first year of marriage, Dana had suffered a complicated, life-threatening miscarriage. Jonathan was on the verge of a nervous breakdown, convinced she was going to die just like his father.

Dana survived, but was told she would never be able to bear children. Adoption was recommended, but the two of them refused to even consider the possibility.

Nurse Hedda had no information for the time after the couple had moved away. I thanked her for the details she had provided. I could now consider the couple's behavior from a fresh perspective.

I had, of course, asked Jonathan several times whether there were any illnesses in his family, but he had firmly denied it and Dana had not corrected him. As for childbearing, I remembered clearly that on their first visit both had professed their disinclination to have children because of their hectic lifestyle and respective careers. I distinctly recalled Dana adding that she felt that there was no justification for bringing children into a violent world such as ours. At the time I had thought that perhaps it was a natural reaction to the terrible wars that Israel had been through. After all, the shock waves of the sudden powerful attacks by Egyptian and Syrian armies in 1973 were still reverberating through all our minds.

Israel is a small country, and almost everyone knew someone who had been killed or wounded in the *Yom Kippur* war. The atmosphere was still charged with grief and bewilderment. A political upheaval had just taken place. For the first time in Israel's short history, the right-wing Likud party under Menachem Begin was elected to rule the country. Everything was in flux. At such times it was not surprising that a couple would decide not to have children.

But nurse Hedda's information pointed me toward further questions. Might their resistance to adoption be a consequence of their defenses to cope with pain? Had they both suppressed the memory of their shared traumas- her miscarriage and his illness?

I began wondering if their protestations about not raising children were another facet of their inability to confront harsh realities. All the rational explanations they had given me at our first meeting of why they were childless now seemed questionable. I could see a source for their refusal to touch on anything that could prove unbearably painful—caring for a child at one end of the spectrum, dealing with a life-threatening disease on the other.

I suppose that every physician reviews his or her actions when faced with an impasse. After all, there was nothing that medicine could offer Jonathan at the time by way of treatment. Hadn't their shared avoidance of pain, their unspoken strategy for survival and success, served them well, better than medicine could? What was my true obligation to them as their physician? Could I have put their right to denial before my responsibility to warn them as best I could? Who was I to deprive them of their shield? For all I knew, this unique bond of theirs, a profound double denial I was never again to encounter in forty years of practice, was precisely what kept them successful and thriving.

Three years after my first encounter with Jonathan and Dana, my wife and I were at the airport waiting to board a flight to London when we suddenly came across the two of them. We exchanged pleasantries and asked where they were going. They were on their way to a rock-climbing holiday in the Dolomites. They had sent all their gear ahead, and they were going directly to the mountain village where they were to start their climbing the following day.

I was horrified. "Is that a good idea?"

"Why not?" Dana smiled serenely. "After all, you found nothing seriously wrong with Jonathan. And you told us we could carry on just as before."

7.

PENANCE

It was David, calling from London. "Could you please see Maya, an employee of mine?"

Chairman of an international advertising conglomerate, David takes close interest in his employees' personal well-being. He has intimate knowledge of their problems and never takes no for an answer in his persistent efforts to offer them assistance.

I couldn't refuse to help a close friend, so I made room in my schedule. David thanked me briskly and was about to hang up.

"Hang on," I stopped him. "At least clue me in as to Maya's problem—some background information, anything on what this is all about."

"It's all about a broken arm that's taking a very long time to heal."

I was surprised. "I'm not an orthopedic specialist, you know that. And there's nothing unusual about a long healing period for fractures."

"We're talking years here. And she's already seen the best orthopedic people in three countries."

"But how can I help? Surely the doctors she's seen are first-class?"

"It's your mind I want on this, not expertise in orthopedics. This is a very special case, and we both know you've always enjoyed a challenge. I'll fly her in to see you tomorrow."

Now I was even more bewildered. "That's ridiculous, David. What is the urgency if it's been going on for years?"

"Believe me, you'll understand when you see her," he said with finality and hung up.

As Maya walked into my office a few days later, I realized immediately that David was right. This was indeed a special case. Maya was a young woman, about thirty years of age, very thin with sharp features, and hair severely tied back into a tight bun. She wore harem pants and a short-sleeved T-shirt, and her right arm nestled in a sling. It looked a bit like a folded bird's wing, held tightly to her body in a strained, unnatural angle. She offered me her left hand to shake as we exchanged hellos.

When she began to speak, unfazed by my ill-concealed scrutiny, she struck me as excessively forceful, perhaps even confrontational. We exchanged a few niceties about her boss. I thought she would be grateful for his concern and efforts on her behalf, but she seemed to coolly accept them as her due. She was one of his best workers, she informed me, so it was only natural he would look out for her when she was ill.

"And are you ill?" I asked, indicating her right arm, which she hadn't moved at all since she came in. I wanted to hear in her own words what she thought the problem was.

"No, not ill at all, just somewhat incapacitated by this thing," she said sarcastically, looking down at her arm in its sling. "I took a fall a couple of years ago and broke a bone in my wrist—the scaphoid bone, they call it—and although they tell me the bone has healed, it just hurts worse and worse. The pain is really unbearable whenever I try to use my hand or even move it, let alone move any part of my arm up to the shoulder. I can't straighten my arm or lift anything. I can't write properly and have to use my left hand. Ordinary painkillers and an endless variety of splints haven't helped at all. And now they're even suggesting doing an operation on my spine, to implant some kind of electrodes that are supposed to stop the pain."

Walking toward the armchair she was seated in, I asked if I could have a look at her arm.

She shrank back, half-turning her right shoulder and arm away from me, and said, "If you must, but be very careful. Every movement hurts like hell." Facing me again, she allowed me to slip the sling over her head and release her arm while supporting it at the elbow.

I could see what a sorry state her whole upper limb was in. She held her arm tightly to her chest wall, from the shoulder joint down. The forearm was bent forward and upward, in severe flexion at the elbow, toward the notch of her neck. The hand was maximally bent at the wrist, the fingers contracted and claw-like. There was no spontaneous movement at all, and when I tried to see if I could elicit any passive movement, she pushed my hands away.

"Oh no! No way are you going to make me move the arm. I've had enough painful manipulations from you doctors to last me a lifetime!" she almost shouted. In a calmer but more assertive tone, she continued, "Look, I don't know what David has been telling you, but the only reason for my being here is to ask for your opinion about all the pain medications they've been pouring into me. How much longer can I go on like this before they make my kidneys rot or give me a heart attack? David says you specialize in drugs and their effects on the body, and that's all I want from you. So can we please get on with that?"

"Certainly," I said, "in a moment. But did you bring your X-rays with you? At least let me have a look at those."

"Of course I did, and you're welcome to see them," she replied tersely. Delving into her large handbag, she produced a brown packet full of X-ray films. I scanned them quickly. I realized I wasn't going to find anything that the British orthopedic specialists had missed. Just as she had reported, her wrist bone had in fact healed quite well within two months of her fall, with no need for surgery. And yet her pain had mounted and spread from the wrist upward to the elbow and shoulder joint, and now it was so severe and so relentless that she could no longer move her right arm and forearm in any direction.

"Oh yes, I brought these too," said Maya, handing me a file of letters and reports from her doctors in London. They were very clear: she was suffering a disorder known as complex regional pain syndrome, or by an older, more commonly used name, reflex sympathetic dystrophy (RSD). This is a condition common in patients recovering from even minimal trauma to a limb or joint, which affects thousands of people every year. It is characterized by constant, progressively worse pain that is neither proportional to the severity of the initial injury (sometimes no worse than a sprain) nor dependent on the healing process. Often it continues unabated long after the originally injured joint or bone has healed completely.

RSD is actually a chronic neurological syndrome, thought to result from malfunctioning of part of the nervous system, with misfired pain signals sent to the brain from the area of the original injury. Left untreated, patients will often develop loss of range of motion and muscle spasms and contractures, leading in extreme cases to total loss of function of the affected limb. Other symptoms include extreme sensitivity to touch, changes in skin color, swelling, and even osteoporosis in the underlying bone structures. Treatment is notoriously difficult in such cases, and there are no magic bullets. It consists mainly of emotional reassurance combined with intensive physiotherapy, and pain control ranging from mild analgesics to the most potent narcotic medications. Sympathetic nerve blockading with injections of local anesthetic is sometimes helpful as well.

More extreme cases may require a sympathectomy, a surgical procedure to sever the sympathetic nerves serving the affected limb. The spinal implantation Maya mentioned is an even more invasive intervention wherein spinal cord stimulators act electrically to dampen the false nerve messages sent to the brain. In the rarest, most severe cases involving crippling pain, joint contractures, muscle atrophy, and irreversible loss of all functional capacity, amputation of the affected limb may remain the last-resort treatment modality.

The intelligent, forceful young woman sitting opposite me had already seen numerous specialists who had been of no help to her. She had heard, digested, and probably regurgitated all this information many times over and was by now an expert on RSD. Aware of how mistrusting she must have become, I decided to ease into the subject, and started out by asking her to tell me how she broke her wrist in the first place.

"I used to devote a good bit of my time to a lot of intensive physical activity. It may be difficult to imagine from looking at me now, but I used to have a nice firm figure, believe it or not. Not like the scarecrow I have become, all skin and bones." She looked down at her body ruefully. "I've always been a sports lover. I played basketball twice a week after work when I lived in Israel, and cycled long distances every weekend. When I moved to the UK, I exchanged basketball for gym and tennis and I was out running in Regent's Park every day, even if it was raining. It was out there, on one of my lunchtime runs, that I fell and broke my wrist bone.

"It really didn't seem a big deal at the time. I went to the hospital, where they told me I'd fractured a small bone in my wrist, put my arm in plaster from the elbow and over the wrist, and said that surgery wouldn't be necessary. It didn't hurt that much, and I was even surprised to learn it was broken. They also said I'd be able to resume running in no time, so I wasn't worried. But then, when they took off the plaster cast six weeks later, this happened." She pointed down at her arm sling.

"Could you elaborate on what you mean by 'this'?" I asked.

"At first there was pain, more than I had felt before. But the doctors said it was natural to still have a bit of pain and recommended that I use ordinary painkillers and exercise the wrist several times a day. I'd soon be as good as new, they promised. I tried, but things just got worse, so I stopped. After a short time, I just couldn't move any part of my arm without experiencing fierce burning pain that would spread upward, from the wrist to the elbow, even to the shoulder."

She broke off and remained silent.

After a few moments, I tried to get her talking again. "What did your doctor tell you about this pain, which was refusing to go away?"

"He said I'd have to exercise the arm constantly despite the pain. Exercising 'into the pain' is what he called it. He explained what RSD was and outlined all its ramifications, saying there was no easy way around it and that I'd have to continue using the arm no matter what. He'd certainly give me a prescription for something stronger for the pain, but I shouldn't expect the pills to work miracles. 'When push comes to shove, dear, it's going to be up to you, and only you'—that's how he put it. 'No one else can do it for you.'"

"Did you follow his advice?"

She threw me an exasperated glance. "Of course. I tried, I really tried, for months and months, but the pain was so bad I eventually decided I'd rather die than exercise into the pain. It was simply impossible to lift my arm more than a few inches.

"I read the leaflets of the pain medications carefully," she continued. "I know they're doing me no good and that in the long run I'm going to ruin something, my stomach or my kidneys or whatnot. But I can't stop. I really hope you can offer me some good advice about these pills and make this trip worthwhile."

"Did you go back to the doctor to tell him all this?" I asked, disregarding her last remark.

"No. I went to another doctor and another and another, and they all said the same thing—exercise into the pain, and the sooner you get on with it the better, before things get even worse. But for me, things couldn't get any worse. Would you call this living? Traveling is out. Even working at my desk is becoming impossible. I can't go out with friends. Even my running partners, who had been very sympathetic and supportive at first, started avoiding me as the lunch hour approached. I could see they felt guilty about running when I obviously couldn't join them. In the end, I simply stopped seeing them altogether. My entire life fell to pieces."

All this was delivered matter-of-factly, with no vocal inflection. Sensing her mounting despair, I wondered if she'd given up on her chances of beating the condition.

"Did you try to do the exercises on your own, or did you go to a professional physiotherapist?" I asked.

"Both. And how. I even participated in group physiotherapy for people with RSD. I was by far the worst case in the class. Anyway, I quickly realized it was doing me no good, so I stopped going."

"Where does David come Into the picture?"

"Well, you know David. He's like a bulldog, and he just wouldn't let go. He sent me to all the specialists he could get hold of. They gave me ganglion blocks by injection and antidepressants and antiepileptic pills that are supposed to be good for that kind of pain but only made me drowsy all day. I also tried acupuncture, ultrasound treatment, electric nerve stimulation, and intravenous infusions of lidocaine. I went to pain clinics, chiropractors, Korean pain massage therapists. Believe me, I've run the whole gamut of treatments, doctors, specialists, and experts. No one has been able to help me. To tell you the truth, no disrespect intended, I'm only here to please David and perhaps find out how best to continue using my painkillers without them killing me first."

David was right. This was indeed a challenge. There seemed to be nothing Maya hadn't tried. Could I offer anything new?

It's been suggested that brain dysfunction may play a role in the underpinnings of the disorder, so that psychological therapy may also be explored in its management. Although antidepressant drugs are standard components of pain treatment, other psychotropic medications or in-depth psychotherapy have not been conclusively proven effective by systematic research. Admittedly, if psychotherapy is to have a meaningful effect, it should be undertaken early on. But in Maya's case, there was nothing to lose by trying it. Better late than never, I thought.

"Have any of your doctors talked to you about looking into possible psychological aspects of your problem, psychotherapy perhaps, to help you deal with your disability and pain?" I asked.

As with so many of my patients the subject of psychotherapy provoked an angry response.

"Of course some did," she snapped. "Some did indeed suggest psychiatric treatment, but I found the suggestion ridiculous. It isn't my mind that's inventing the pain. It's really there, and it's really terrible.

No amount of psychological mumbo jumbo will take it away. I've often thought that if any of you doctors who were offering this advice were to experience anything as harrowing as my pain, you wouldn't make such silly suggestions."

Her extreme reaction baffled me. It is well known that physical pain is often compounded by emotional distress. And yet this obviously intelligent person was completely unreceptive to the notion. Neither the radical disproportion between her paralyzing pain and its modest source nor her failure to "work into the pain," disciplined though she was, suggested to her there might be psychological factors at work. But resistance to treatment of conditions potentially treatable by medical methods does require looking into such factors. Since open discussion of psychotherapeutic options was clearly out of the question, I opted for an indirect approach.

"I'm sorry if I've upset you," I said, "but you really haven't told me much about yourself."

Maya readily launched into a detailed description of David's organization and her highly responsible position in it. "You wouldn't believe how many people I supervise in our marketing division and what it takes to keep them on track. We have milestones to meet, you know, and if we don't, some of them are going to be out of a job. The hours I put in, day and night—if it weren't for my lunchtime running, I think I'd go crazy. I haven't had a decent holiday in—"

"No," I interrupted her. "I meant about *yourself*, your family perhaps, or where you grew up and went to school. David told me that in your military service you were one of the first girls to qualify as a weapons instructor for new recruits. Tell me about that, or why you left home, or how you ended up living in London."

No response. She became very still. She just wouldn't talk about herself.

Something in her defiant demeanor, so much in contrast with her evident despair and helplessness, led me to try a different tack. Resuming the role she had cast me in—a physician with drug expertise—I decided to move to more neutral ground.

"Other than your arm, how is your health, generally speaking?" I asked. "Are there any other medical problems bothering you now? Have you had any serious health issues in the past?"

"No, I haven't had any illnesses since childhood," she answered. "As a kid, I think I contracted every childhood illness under the sun." For the first time in our talk, she smiled. "They used to put my little sister into my bed, hoping that she too would catch the chicken pox or measles or mumps or whatever I was down with, so that we'd both be immune in later life. But she never managed to get infected and went blissfully through childhood without a single bout of illness."

"Where does your sister live?"

She stiffened.

"In Israel. Until recently she lived with my mother—in the same house, actually, where we both grew up. But she got married and moved to another area of greater Tel Aviv."

Her voice, I noticed, had become tenser as she spoke of her sister.

"What about your mother?" I asked. "Does she live alone now?"

"I'm afraid so. My father died a few years ago. My mother became very depressed and withdrawn, and my sister volunteered to go on living at home with her. This made it possible for me to leave Israel and go to London, something I had always wanted to do. With her there, my mother was able to function somehow, but her depression just got worse, and she started recounting endless memories of all her past troubles." Maya paused. "She even started talking about the death camps in Europe, which we two had never heard her speak of, ever."

"What's going to happen now that your sister has married and moved out?"

"I don't know," Maya said. "My mother can't be left alone and refuses to have someone move in with her. Won't have a stranger roaming around her house disrupting her routine. She says she'd rather die."

I noticed that Maya's left hand had taken hold of her right wrist, gripping it tightly.

"I take it your mother is a Holocaust survivor. Did you just say that she and your father never spoke of the Holocaust with you and your sister?"

"That's right," she said. "They never did. Growing up, my sister and I were different from our friends. We had no family stories to tell, no grandparents, no pictures of aunts or uncles or cousins, nothing. Just the four of us, until my father died. That was when my mother first opened up. They were from Germany. They didn't get out in time. Somehow, they stayed alive. They were rounded up in one of the deportations to the camps and separated immediately, finding themselves on different trains but in the same kind of cattle cars.

"My mother ended up in Ravensbruck, my father in Mauthausen. She played the piano for the SS officers. He was a shoemaker and ended up polishing their boots and fixing soles and heels. Both of them worked for some extra crusts of bread or potato peels. Somehow, they both survived. It was truly a miracle that they were reunited in a DP camp in Italy in 1946. When they tried to get to Palestine on one of the illegal immigrant ships, they were intercepted by the British and interned in a camp on Cyprus for another eighteen months. Isn't it ironic that I've found myself living in London?"

"What language did you speak at home?" I asked.

"Only Hebrew. Although the subject was always avoided, we knew somehow that they had come from Germany, but it was forbidden to speak German in the house."

This was not unusual. The self-imposed silence of the survivors was well known in the Israel of the 1950s. Many of these ravaged people refused to talk about any of their experiences, unable as they were to deal with the emotional wounds. Some developed severe psychiatric illnesses and required long-term hospitalization. I had met such unfortunate people when I worked as a male nurse in a mental institution in Jerusalem during my medical school years. These encounters were not easily forgotten.

Other survivors, like Maya's parents, perhaps stronger of spirit, went on to create new lives. When children of these Holocaust survivors—the second generation, as they were called in later years—were interviewed, they described their parents' silence as a heavy shadow cast over the household. Some characterized it as depressing; others used terms like "disturbing" or "threatening." All spoke of a sense of great pain.

Outside the house, however, life went on for these children. They grew up, went to school, served in the army, and attended university. In recent years some of them have written autobiographical novels, which have been widely read in Israel. Their stories often revolve around their generation's sense of guilt for preferring not to know, for their relief at not having to share their parents' painful memories.

Was Maya one of those children of silence? Growing up, she did not know, was not allowed to know, of her mother's suffering. There was no number tattooed on her mother's arm (tattoos were done only at Auschwitz) and no other hint of the ordeal. Could the void she had grown up with, her possible willing ignorance and the guilt it engendered, be somehow related to her present suffering? Or perhaps her flight to the UK, far from the responsibilities of caring for her aging mother, was born of dismay, or even anger, at her mother's lifelong silence? Yet how could one be angry at Holocaust survivors? Was this, perhaps, another source of guilt? And now she was still tucked away in London, taking no part in her mother's suffering. Could her relentless pain syndrome and inability to help herself be symptomatic of such inner turmoil?

"Does your sister feel you should come back to Israel and take over the care of your mother?" I asked.

"Well, she doesn't say so in so many words, but it's obvious to me she thinks I'm selfish in not coming back. After all, she did look after my mother when I went off to pursue my career, and now I'm sure she expects me to do the same for her." Maya spoke tensely, avoiding eye contact and directing her gaze at a fixed point on the wall behind my desk

"How do you feel about the idea of coming back to Israel?"

Maya fidgeted, still not looking at me. "I can't possibly go back until I'm well again. My sister doesn't understand I'm truly ill, in constant pain, and unable to take care of myself, let alone my mother."

"Do you have friends in Israel?"

"Not many. I haven't kept up relations with them. There isn't much point, is there? Why should they seek my company any more than my British friends, who feel sorry for me but avoid me like the plague? No one wants someone else's pain inflicted on them."

"What does your mother say about all this?" I asked.

"Oh, she maintains a thunderous silence. Every time I phone, she answers my questions but never volunteers a word of her own. She never asks how I am. She doesn't ask me to come back. On the contrary, she always says she doesn't need anybody and can manage fine on her own."

"Does she know about your condition? Have you ever discussed it with her?"

"No point, she'd only say it's all psychological. And she'd see my inability to cope with the pain as a weakness that is not to be tolerated. After all, she has been through the worst experiences imaginable and survived, so why would she understand or sympathize with what I'm going through?"

By now there were tears in Maya's eyes, and her forcefulness was gone. I had a first glimpse of her deep sadness, and it strengthened my conviction that her state of mind could well be a major factor in her complicated physical disability. I wondered what I could offer her that had not already been suggested. But I needed to find out just how bad things were.

"Would you allow me to complete my examination of your arm?" I asked.

The tears were gone now, and she was back to her self-assured, defiant stance. "What's the point? We both know that there's no cure for my condition. Why waste your time and mine with useless examinations?"

"Well, since you've taken the trouble of flying in from England specifically for this appointment, I think another few minutes of your time and mine would not be out of order. Naturally, I'm confident that the doctors who examined you in the UK did not miss anything, but I really could not give you my considered opinion about your illness without examining you properly myself. I'm sure that in your own work you're just as thorough and check everything out for yourself."

The reference to her professionalism proved helpful, for she agreed to let me examine her again. I asked her to show me the degree to which she could move her arm in different directions, but she couldn't comply. As before, my attempts to elicit passive movements at the shoulder or elbow joints were unsuccessful, but I felt that now she was making an effort to cooperate with my examination, which clearly caused her a lot of pain.

It took no time at all, nor great perception, to realize that her condition was very advanced. Due to the long disuse and lack of motion, her large muscle groups were atrophied and the shoulder, elbow, and wrist were in fixed contractures, with no motion possible of this folded, wing like appendage. With the wrist tightly flexed too, the small muscles of her hand were also atrophied, the fingers bent into a talon-like position which the French call *main en griffe*.

I now realized full well that the time lapse since the injury and the total immobility of the limb had led to anatomical and functional changes that at this stage may well have been irreversible.

We had been together for over an hour when I recalled her doctors' recommendation of spinal cord stimulation by implanted electrodes. Given the failure of all other means of pain control, they said, this last-resort measure, combined with concentrated physiotherapy for the arm, might offer some improvement. I too felt that intensive activation of the arm by all available means was the only hope of breaking the vicious cycle of pain and disuse. But I also felt that psychological intervention would have to precede any physical procedure, particularly surgery, if the latter were to succeed. Was there any way to overcome her resistance to psychologists, psychotherapy, psychiatrists, and the lot?

I then remembered a patient of mine, a personal friend, who had come to see me a few years before in despair. A vital, healthy sixty-five-year-old, he was an avid tennis player. During one game he tripped and severely sprained his ankle. After fractured bones and torn ligaments were ruled out, he was put in a plaster cast for six weeks. Following its removal, he developed much the same syndrome as that afflicting Maya. Trying to resume his normal activities, he found he experienced more and more pain. He stopped putting weight on his foot, adopted a shuffling gait, and couldn't walk without a cane. A bone scan had revealed some inflammation around the ankle joint for which he received local cortisone-like injections and large doses of analgesics, to no avail. By the time he came to me, five months had already elapsed since the injury and he had given up trying. Like Maya, he too had been told to work into the pain, but soon he just couldn't bear it.

And like Maya, this confident, self-assured man had sat across from me totally helpless, insisting there was no way he could deal with the pain incurred by practicing walking on the injured ankle. But in his case it wasn't too hard to get through to him. Having known him for years as something of a dandy, very particular about his appearance and fitness, I simply appealed to his vanity.

"Look at you, hobbling along on your stick like an old man," I'd said to him. "And it's only going to get worse. I really think you're not ready to have people think of you as such. Neither am I, and I'm willing to help. Let's start right here and now!"

It took six long sessions of walking up and down my office rug without a cane to persuade him to continue making the effort on his own. Finally, he did. It was an excruciatingly difficult experience, but he persevered and very slowly improved. Today he is walking normally. In winter he even skis, though very carefully. Sometimes the pain comes back, but he walks through it. In his case, all it took was an appeal to his strong sense of self-image, a challenge to his masculinity perhaps. Maya, I knew, was in a different league altogether—not a case for simple common sense and a bit of friendly badgering. Still, it occurred to me that if she was to meet my friend, she might see that recovery was possible, no matter how bad her despair. However, when I suggested the idea, she contemptuously refused.

"No, I've already tried that. Remember I told you I had been to RSD group treatment in the UK? That didn't help, so why would a former patient of yours? That's just old hat. All you physicians offer the same old bag of tricks. You don't really know how to treat this disorder, do you? Why don't you just admit it?" She got up to go.

"I will admit that there is no one way to treat this disorder," I said. "It has many manifestations, and different treatments work for different people. In your case, I would definitely recommend enlisting the help of a psychotherapist to help you deal with the pain. I would not give up if I were you, because you have everything to lose and nothing to gain by giving up. I realize you're disillusioned by where you've gotten so far, but I recommend fighting on. You seem to me to be a fighter, and I believe you can do it."

I said these words as she reached the door. She did not turn around.

Later that week David called to thank me for seeing Maya. I told him I felt I had failed miserably with her.

"Not so," he said. "She has come back and actually told me that you admitted you didn't know anything about her disorder. In fact, she accused you of proposing the same old junk that all the others had proposed." However, he chuckled, Maya had started seeing a psychotherapist.

I was extremely happy to hear that I had made a slight dent in her armor. I asked David to keep me posted on her progress.

The story, however, did not have a happy ending. About a year later, David informed me that Maya's condition had deteriorated terribly. She had the spinal electrodes procedure, which did no good. The pain got so bad she needed injections of morphine. In the end, the arm had to be amputated. She was now in rehabilitation, learning to adapt to a prosthetic arm, and gradually being weaned from the opiates she had become addicted to.

Thinking back on Maya's story, I am left feeling deeply frustrated. I have tried to analyze our interaction time and again. I think of what she said and how she said it and try to understand what she had left unsaid. I review her body language, her aggressive stance, her hostile resistance to me, her expression of contempt for all doctors, and I try to reassure myself that this did not get in the way of my efforts to break down the barriers she had erected. Was her disengagement from her mother's suffering, past and present, really the root of her problem, and was her torment a kind of penance?

I do not believe this is the whole story and feel there is a lot more undisclosed, pushed deep beneath the surface I had reached with my probing. I try to console myself with the reasoning that she was so far gone by the time she reached me that she was really beyond help. But then I ask myself whether I might have been able to help her try to overcome the disability she embraced so tightly had I been able to feel her unspoken language. But, on the other hand, perhaps not. There are, after all, barriers in communication that, even if recognized by the physician, cannot be surmounted.

As so often happens in rethinking these stories, I feel the bitter sadness of failure.

8.

SHUTTERED LISTENERS

I first met Alice at a dinner in her honor at the home of her daughter and son-in-law.

Pam and Ben Stein were English. They had originally been sent to Israel by Ben's company on a two-year assignment but had fallen in love with the country and decided to stay. Ben was an engineer presently employed by an Israeli outfit specializing in conveyor belts for airports; Pam was a successful writer of mystery novels set against an Israeli backdrop. They had moved into our neighborhood six months earlier, and we had become very close friends. Ben was open, outgoing, and always cheerful, while Pam was reserved, quiet, and thoughtful. She had often spoken of her mother, whom we had never met. Pam's father had died some years earlier. Although her mother had totally relied on him for everything in life and never had to fend for herself, it seemed, according to the stories Pam related from time to time, that her mother had smoothly shed her helplessness. She had emerged as an independent, totally self-sufficient social butterfly, moving from one party to the next in London and Tel Aviv and traveling round the world on cruises to exotic places. I was curious to meet her, expecting quite a character, if Pam's descriptions were anything to go by.

I found Alice to be a formidable lady, indeed, whose appearance was striking, elegant, vivacious, and youthful. She prided herself on looking far less than her sixty years. She dominated the dinner table effortlessly with sparkling descriptions of people she had met, art exhibitions she had recently seen, and new books she had just read. It was clear that she tended to lay down the law and was critical of other people's tastes that did not agree with her own. She was somehow overenthusiastic about plays she had seen or "important" paintings she liked. She used superlatives that left no room for disagreement. "The best I've ever seen" and "the most fantastic ever performed," she pronounced, dismissing any potential opposition imperiously. Notwithstanding a certain sense of irritation, I found her intelligent, interesting to talk to, and a good dinner companion. She really did know a lot, cared very much about the arts, and had a natural curiosity about everything around her. I also noticed, however, that she didn't show much interest in the mundane—children, grandchildren, life in Israel, politics.

It was also clear that Pam was under considerable tension during the dinner, which was especially discernible whenever she served the various courses to her mother. I was surprised. Pam's culinary prowess was famous, and she was usually completely relaxed about her cooking. It was when her mother failed to compliment her on her cooking and refused second helpings that I realized this must have been a longstanding issue between them. Later, after Alice had left, Pam suddenly exploded in a veritable torrent of angry recrimination against her mother. This was very unusual for someone so reserved and private. I realized then that this was a deep-rooted emotion, for her mother had done nothing that I could see that evening to bring on such an outburst of uncontrolled resentment and pain.

"She's the only person in the world who doesn't like my cooking," said Pam, almost in tears. "She never likes anything I serve. She objects to the way I lay the table. She disapproves of the things I wear. She doesn't like the way I do my hair. In fact, she has never approved of anything I've done. She has been critical of everything and anything ever since I can remember, and I have never managed to please her.

"As a child I remember saving up for months to buy her a cigarette box for her birthday. When I presented it to her expectantly with great pride, she looked at it unenthusiastically. 'Thank you, dear.' It was never used or even seen again. Can you imagine what that felt like to an eight-year-old? Since then, birthday after birthday, the pattern repeated itself. Watches, bags, jewelry, scarves—all followed the cigarette box into oblivion. Today I no longer buy her presents for her birthday, but even the flowers I send her are never to her taste. She never comments on them directly, but a few months later on the appropriate occasion, she'll say something like, 'I hope you made sure that the flowers you sent so-and-so were nicer than those the shop sent me on my birthday.'"

A lot of bitterness came pouring out. It seemed as though forty years of maternal dismissal had suddenly been crystallized for Pam by the friction at the dinner table.

Ben went to get her a drink. The outburst obviously did not come as a surprise to him. He had heard it all before and took it with his usual equanimity.

"Have you ever tried talking to your mother about all this?" I asked Pam, trying to calm her down.

"There's no point. Whenever I tried discussing it with her, she would answer, 'Well, dear, I always tell the truth about aesthetics. You surely wouldn't want me to lie to you?' She has convinced herself that aesthetics are holy and her understanding of them infallible. So I gave up trying long ago. Sometimes I still feel like that eight-year-old child."

Pam calmed down and we left quickly, before she could regret her outburst in our presence.

During her stay in Israel, I saw Alice quite a few times at the Steins' home. On one of these occasions, she mentioned that she had a strange "heart condition" that doctors in the UK had not been able to diagnose for many years. When I asked her for more details, she shrugged it off. "Talking about one's health is just too boring," she said, launching immediately into an exuberant description of a lecture she had just attended on the influence of postwar German artists on modern Israeli painting.

Pam, however, confirmed that her mother had indeed been suffering from unexplained irregular heartbeats for as long as she could remember. "I myself witnessed countless onsets of these 'attacks,' and they were always quite frightening. My mother would suddenly be covered in sweat, or as she always corrected, 'Perspiration, dear. Ladies perspire; they do not sweat.' Feeling lightheaded, she would have to find somewhere to sit down, which was not always easy, especially if we happened to be on the street or in a busy department store. The attack would last only a few minutes, and then she'd be back to herself, and we would continue whatever we were doing as though nothing had happened," Pam recalled.

"My mother could never bear anyone seeing her in that state and always put on a show for anyone who happened to be passing, pretending that all was well and that she was just resting. If anyone stopped to ask what was wrong, she always answered, 'My dear, what could possibly be wrong?' She is an expert at denying anything unpleasant. Her theory is that if you don't talk about the unpleasant things of life, they will just go away. Her brother is a schizophrenic, but my mother has always maintained that he was just slightly eccentric. Her own mother suffered from senile dementia and had to be put in an old-age home, where she stayed for many years until the end of her life. But my mother has always maintained that there was nothing wrong with my grandmother, and that she was in the old-age home for just a few days before she died peacefully."

"But surely, even people who deny unpleasant things usually seek medical attention for the kind of symptoms you have described?" I asked.

"Oh, she has been to see more than one cardiologist in London and has had every possible test done, including a heart-rhythm monitor, to which she was hooked up repeatedly. All these tests came up negative. She was told over and over that all she had were bouts of sinus tachycardia, fast—but normal—heartbeats, probably brought on by anxiety. She wasn't happy about the diagnosis and has always insisted that they were wrong."

"What do you think?" I asked.

"I think they were probably right. After all, we are talking of the very best specialists in the UK. Surely they can't all be wrong? It's been going on for forty years or so and hasn't gotten worse. She is neurotic, and in any case there's not much that we can do about it. Besides, she has learned to live with it, so perhaps it's best left alone."

Alice went back to England, and it was some time before I saw her again, on her next visit to Israel. She looked well and was full of beans as always, very much sought after, especially, as she never failed to remind all of us, by younger people of our age. She embarked on a whirlwind round of social visits, which she soundly enjoyed, moving all over the country. Jerusalem in the morning, Tel Aviv in the evening, and a game of bridge in between. Her parties were famous. My wife and I were invited to some of them. Unlike the usual Israeli style of plying guests with an enormous selection of food, she believed in small portions of delicacies and lots of vodka to create a good mood. She wasn't going to bow to any local form of entertaining.

"I have my own style, and anyone who doesn't like it can just stay home," she tartly informed us. Her energy was simply astounding, and her self-confidence supreme.

One afternoon, however, she phoned and asked me to come to Tel Aviv to see her. She asked me not to talk to Pam and Ben about it, as she didn't want to worry them unduly. She received me in her beautiful penthouse, dressed in a fine Chinese silk dressing gown and high-heeled slippers. Instead of the usual marble or ceramic floors found in Israel, here a soft, deep-piled carpet in apricot stretched from wall to wall over the whole apartment. The dainty crystals of a French chandelier hung over an Italian, pale-gray marble table surrounded by black cane chairs. For a moment I thought that she really belonged to another time and another place. The image of a nineteenth-century salon somewhere in Europe came to mind, with its mellow colors and soft lighting. She seemed to be out of place in the harsh Mediterranean light, which, incidentally, she took great care to keep out with the aid of cream linen curtains.

But then I looked around her spacious but sparingly furnished living room and was overwhelmed by the strong blues, reds, and yellows bursting from the canvases on the walls. "These are mostly early twentieth-century German expressionists," she explained, noticing my amazement. The subtly lit sculptures and other contemporary works of art displayed round the room also strongly stated her taste for the modern. I revised my first impression. Strangely enough, she really seemed to span both worlds.

My tea arrived in a silver Georgian teapot accompanied by tiny chestnut truffles on a matching silver dish.

Settling down on the white sofa with a glass of whiskey in her hand, Alice proceeded to tell me that she'd had two of her attacks in the past twenty-four hours. "I'm beginning to be anxious about the situation," she said. "My heartbeats have become more violent in the past few weeks. I didn't want to give up any of my activities—I have a lot on this week, you see—so I decided to fortify myself with whiskey and continued as planned. But now things are getting worse. Can you give me something to stop these violent attacks?"

"Why don't we start with you telling me exactly what you feel when you get these attacks?" I said.

"Well, you know already," she answered. "I get these attacks of tachycardia and malaise."

"No, no, I don't want you to use medical jargon. I want you to simply describe for me, in detail, exactly how these attacks come on, the sequence of your symptoms, your sensations."

"I *am* telling you what I feel. I feel an arrhythmia coming on."

I tried again. "Please do not use medical terms. Just describe in plain language what you feel. It is very important for me to get a sense of what you are experiencing rather than what you've been told you are experiencing."

She was indignant. "You do not realize I am not simply repeating what the doctors have told me. I have a medical encyclopedia next to my bed, which I often consult. I have read a lot about my disorder, and although you obviously consider me an uninformed layman, I think I am qualified to use medical terms."

"Nonetheless, I am asking you to put aside what you have read and what you have been told and simply describe in everyday language what you feel when one of these attacks comes on," I said as patiently as I could.

Though apparently offended by my lack of appreciation for her medical learning, Alice grudgingly did as she was told but still sprinkled her tale with terms such as "malaise" or a "nearly fainting syncope-like sensation." When she saw that I was getting impatient, she moved to a more precise description.

"I feel my heart beating very fast. I actually hear it drumming in my ears. I feel out of breath, and then I begin to perspire. My head gets light, and I feel that I am about to lose consciousness, although that has never in fact happened. I have had it for so many years that I have become used to it, but it is getting worse."

"When did it all start?" I asked.

"Oh, it was really a long time ago, probably in my thirties. I was driving a car all alone when I suddenly felt my heart pumping and had some difficulty in breathing. I stopped the car, absolutely terrified, convinced I was having a heart attack. A few minutes passed, and the rapid beating stopped, but I couldn't drive; I was too scared. I left the car and took a taxi home. Our family physician, Dr. Solomon, came at once and gave me a thorough examination. He couldn't find anything unusual. He sent me to have an electrocardiogram the next day. Nothing significant showed up. Dr. Solomon then decided on a series of blood tests and X-rays, but all came back negative.

"He then called my husband and me to his office and proceeded to explain that there was nothing wrong with my heart. If indeed there were episodes of rapid heartbeat, something that had yet to be proved, these were probably an expression of anxiety attacks. He explained that these often mimicked heart attacks and that I really needed a psychologist rather than a cardiologist to help me overcome this very unpleasant disorder."

"And did you follow his advice and seek the help of a psychologist?" I asked.

"Of course not. I knew then, as I do now, that my symptoms originate from a real physical disorder that has nothing to do with my mind. Solomon was a good doctor, but in my case, he failed. He just didn't know what was wrong with me, so he took the easy way out, blaming it on some kind of neurosis. I stopped seeing him after he behaved very badly toward me."

"What did he do?" I asked.

"Well, it was when I got an attack in the middle of the night. I really thought I was going to die; it was one of the worst I had ever had. My husband phoned Solomon at three o'clock in the morning and asked him to come. In England it is not customary to call a doctor at night, but he came anyway. I think he realized how scared my husband was, and he was basically a nice man. He did an ECG, which again showed nothing out of the ordinary. He then angrily told us that if I chose to ignore his advice about seeing a psychologist, he would suggest we find another doctor. He left, refusing payment, and that was the last I saw of him. It was a shame, because he was a good doctor for the children, and I liked him." Alice shook her head ruefully as if sorry for poor old Dr. Solomon who had lost her as a patient.

After that episode she went on having attacks, but by now she was used to them and no longer thought she was going to die. So she would find somewhere to sit when they occurred and wait for them to pass, which they always did. Occasionally, she went to see this well-known cardiologist or that highly recommended internist, but the result was always the same. Her problem was psychosomatic. All tests were negative. There was nothing there.

I asked to see her test reports, but she did not have them with her. She had left them in England but would bring them next time she came to Israel. I examined her and found nothing out of the ordinary. I must admit that I was inclined to share Dr. Solomon's opinion that she was indeed suffering from anxiety attacks.

And yet something in her personality did not seem to fit that assessment. I couldn't quite put my finger on what it was that didn't seem right, but it was enough to keep me thinking about it. So a few days later, hearing she was due to depart for London once more, I called and went to see her again. She was in fine fettle and kept me talking about some great Spanish painter whom the world had just discovered.

"How have you been feeling?" I asked.

"I feel fine, except for the occasional attack, but I don't let them stop me from doing everything I want to do."

I had been thinking a lot about her, troubled by a thought that had occurred to me right at the beginning, when she first told me her story. I was thinking of a rather uncommon disorder called pheochromocytoma that, if it were the case, could explain many of her symptoms. The pheo (as we called it in diminutive) is a benign tumor that usually grows in the adrenal gland, sitting on top of one of the kidneys. What makes it nasty is that periodically, and in an unheralded fashion, it secretes abnormal quantities of adrenaline (the fight-or-flight hormone produced by the normal adrenal gland in appropriate response to externally or internally induced stress). These spurts of adrenaline pumped into the bloodstream produce classic symptoms—rapid heartbeat, perspiration, changes in blood pressure—often mimicking those of anxiety attacks. Every medical student is taught to think of pheo whenever investigating a patient with transient rises in blood pressure and/or palpitations, or in cases in which anxiety or panic attacks are being considered. Rises in blood pressure were conspicuous by their absence from Alice's medical records. But then again, she had never been observed by a physician during an attack.

At the time, pheo could be diagnosed only by testing the patient's urine for chemical products of the breakdown in the body of the excess adrenaline produced by the tumor. This was best achieved by testing over the hours, or day, following an attack. However, as attacks were usually unpredictable, this was often impractical. The alternative would be to do random, spot urine collections, hoping to catch abnormal adrenaline excretion, even without the presence of symptoms, as often occurred. I couldn't believe that the possibility of pheochromocytoma had not been eliminated long ago in the course of the tests that she had taken.

"Were you ever asked to collect your urine for several hours or overnight or maybe for a whole day?" I asked her.

"No, I don't think so. But I may have forgotten."

As she was leaving Israel again the next day, I decided to write a letter to her doctor in London, on the off chance that the test had not been done. Not wishing to offend him by offering unsolicited advice, I wrote very tactfully that I was sure the test for pheo had indeed been done but perhaps should be repeated several times, just to be on the safe side. I gave Alice the letter to take back with her and advised her against putting off her visit to him. There was no feedback from London, and I assumed that all was well.

She returned to Tel Aviv in early spring, looking well and full of energy as usual.

"What did the GP have to say about my letter?" I asked.

Quite out of character, she fidgeted uneasily. "Actually, he was quite annoyed. Said something about young Israeli know-it-all doctors seeking rare diseases where there were none. He said that he had been in practice for fifty years and had never come across a pheo. Also, he had been looking after me for twenty years and no one was going to tell him what was wrong with me. My disorder was entirely psychosomatic, and there was nothing more to be done." Alice looked embarrassed. "But he did file it in my medical record," she said comfortingly.

I was surprised and even angry. This was not what common professional courtesy prescribed. I would have expected at least a brief reply to my letter.

"In that case, I would like you to do this test here in Israel, just to be on the safe side," I said.

She demurred. "I'm too busy this week. My calendar is absolutely full. We can think about it again next week or the week after."

I couldn't convince her; she was a very stubborn lady.

A couple of weeks passed. Then one evening she phoned to tell me she had been experiencing very bad back pain for three days. She had never had any back pain before and was stunned by its severity.

"You know that I can stand pain very well. I never even have an injection at the dentist. But this is simply awful," she complained.

"Why didn't you call me earlier?" I asked.

"I didn't want to bother you because you live out of town, so I called in a local neurologist that my friends recommended. They all said that he was fantastic at dealing with back pain. He seemed a nice young man, very sure of himself. He promised me that the pain-killer he would inject into my back would alleviate the pain in a matter of minutes."

"And did it?" I asked.

"Unfortunately, it doesn't seem to have helped at all. I think he was overly optimistic," said Alice.

I told her I would be in to see her the next morning, but late that night I was awakened by the phone. It was her maid. Alice was very ill; she had nearly fainted trying to get out of bed, but she was refusing to let the maid call an ambulance, so could I come immediately? I rushed to Tel Aviv and found Alice prostrate, her pulse racing and barely palpable. She was extremely pale and unresponsive. Realizing that there was no time to lose, we literally carried her to my car, and, keeping my hand on the horn, I drove through all the red lights to the hospital.

Our initial examination revealed that although seemingly in shock, her blood pressure was high at 185/100. Her pulse was now down to 95, but it was still fast. There was some tenderness over her lower back, on the right, but no other findings from her physical. Her skin, which had been pale, cold, and clammy, was now warmer, pink, and dry. She was now fully aware of her surroundings and able to respond to questions.

"Something is seriously wrong," she said dryly, echoing my own feeling that what we had just been through was the harbinger of things to come. The elevated blood pressure was the clue. It was what had been missing all along. Pheochromocytoma characteristically causes paroxysms of high blood pressure and sweating palpitations. I was now sure that I had been right. I didn't understand the back pain at that moment, but I knew what had to be done.

At the time, I was a senior physician in the department of medicine at our hospital. My ward was completely full, so Alice was admitted to the adjoining one. Despite the late hour, I phoned the ward chief, Dr. Harry Baum, to put him in the picture. He arrived at the hospital at about the same time as Pam and Ben, whom I had also called and alerted to the situation. I took a few minutes to calm them down and then went back to discuss the case with Dr. Baum.

I briefly recounted the whole story, my interpretation, and tentative diagnosis, and suggested we immediately start the urine collection for testing the next morning. There were also two more urgent to-dos. Treatment had to be started immediately using an intravenous medication called phentolamine to specifically block the effects of the excess adrenaline flowing throughout her body, which, if left untreated, could certainly damage vital organs over the next few hours. We also had to schedule an invasive X-ray procedure called an aortic angiogram as soon as possible to specifically identify and localize the pheo and enable the surgeon to accurately plan the operation for its removal. This was before the time of ultrasound and computed tomography, and the angiogram too was not routinely done, requiring preparation of personnel and equipment.

Almost out of breath, I finished my assessment and suggestions for immediate treatment. But to my amazement, Baum and his deputy, who had also arrived meanwhile, dismissed my analysis out of hand.

"I don't agree with your hypothesis. There are far more common explanations for her condition. I think it's much more likely that she has a bloodstream bacterial infection. We need to draw blood cultures and then start treatment with intravenous fluids and antibiotics. In the morning we will reassess the situation," he said brusquely, getting up to leave.

"What about collecting urine for pheo testing?" I asked.

"All right, although I don't think it's necessary. But that's it. No targeted drug therapy or invasive radiology until we understand the situation better," he said and left the ward.

Baum was a physician of the old European guard, having studied in Budapest and trained in internal medicine in Vienna before escaping to Palestine in 1938. He had been my teacher, and we had often disagreed, even clashed, while I was doing my residency in his department. He was the kind of chief physician who did not take kindly to any kind of argument. His word was law, his experience greater than that of his students and doctors in training, entitling him to insist on things being done his way, unquestioned. He was indeed an excellent doctor—thorough, experienced, and attentive. He took his patients seriously, worked hard, and read widely. He was also inflexible and touchy, taking any expression of disagreement as an insulting hint of mistrust. His sensitivity, I suspected, was rooted in his personal life history.

Our affiliation to the newly established university medical school a few years earlier had found many of the older clinicians unprepared for the "publish or perish" culture of academic appointments. Baum had devoted his entire career to patient care, had not done any research, and had published only a few clinical reports in the medical literature. So he was not awarded the rank of professor. My promotion to that rank at a relatively young age had irritated him. I suppose no one takes kindly to those they regard as young upstarts in the hierarchy. He didn't like my proposals, which I had had the temerity to express at our general medicine meetings, to modernize our clinical methods, introduce more open discussion, rely on more evidence in the literature rather than on anecdotal experience, and listen more attentively to the young house-staff doctors. All this he regarded as too revolutionary, and it was clearly the foundation for much of his resentment.

I can see all this now in hindsight, but at the time I was simply stunned, and very angry. I was quite sure that my analysis and planned course of action were right. Any further delay could be seriously harmful. I could not understand how Baum had ignored my suggestions and not embarked immediately upon their implementation. I stayed with Alice alongside Matthew Ofer, the young resident on duty. Matthew was a bright young doctor about to specialize in cardiology but still at the stage of residency in general medicine. He had witnessed the altercation and—perhaps because he was of the younger and more open-minded generation—had come down firmly on my side.

Over the first hours, Alice remained stable and clear-minded, noting that her back pain had subsided. But suddenly, at two o'clock in the morning, her blood pressure rose to 195/110, her pulse racing at 130. Her skin once more became pale, cold, and clammy. She weakly complained of a new pain in her right lower abdomen.

"Please do something," she whispered. "I feel as if I can't hold out much longer."

"Set up the phentolamine drip immediately," I told Matthew and went off to phone Dr. Baum. Describing the developments, I informed him of what I was doing and said that if he objected, he'd have to come in and take over her management at the bedside, as she was slipping, and fast.

"No," he growled, "you take over, and we'll deal with the way you are behaving in my ward in the morning." The phone went dead in my hand.

It was now three o'clock in the morning. Without further ado I phoned our radiology specialist and told him the entire story. He agreed immediately to perform the angiogram in three hours' time. I also alerted our consulting chief surgeon, asking him to rework his schedule, as we would probably need him to operate at about eight thirty. He too immediately concurred, thrilled by the uniqueness of the story. Upon my return to Alice's bedside, I found Matthew grinning.

"You were right!" he exclaimed.

While I was on the phone, the IV drip of phentolamine had been running for about forty-five minutes. By now her blood pressure was down to 155/85, and her pulse was steady at 98.

"Her skin is regaining its normal color," he said "but I'm beginning to worry about her abdomen."

Alice smiled wanly.

"Sorry to be such a nuisance," she said, "but I do have this different gnawing pain in my belly."

Indeed, the right lower abdomen was tender and tense.

"I am not sure of what is happening in there," I said. "But we will soon know. I'm sure that in a few hours you will be going into surgery to have your pheochromocytoma removed. But first we have to locate it accurately."

I described the angiogram procedure, which involved pushing a catheter through a skin puncture up through her femoral artery (in the groin) into her main abdominal artery, the aorta, and then injecting a radio opaque dye and taking serial X-rays as it coursed through her abdominal organs, outlining them and enabling visualization of their structure, including any abnormality. She took all this in stoically.

"Just get it all going," she said.

Matthew and I watched over her for the next two hours. She was doing splendidly. As the phentolamine dripped in, her blood pressure was steady and so was her pulse. She had weathered the adrenaline storm, I thought, but I remained worried about what we would find when the abdomen was opened. We wheeled her gurney into the angiography room at seven o'clock that morning just as her bag of collected urine was rushed off to the lab.

By eight o'clock it all came together. The X-rays showed a large mass, 8 x 4 cm, sitting on top of her right kidney where her adrenal gland should have been. They also showed leakage of the dye into the tissues around the mass in her lower back. It was now all clear. Her back pain was caused by a hemorrhage, a spontaneous bleed into the large pheochromocytoma that had ruptured, with blood leaking into the surroundings of the inner side of her lower back. This explained the excruciating pain she had felt over the preceding days.

Luckily, the amount of blood collecting in the tissues of her lower back had not been large enough to lead to the consequences of blood loss per se. However, the rupture of the tumor and hemorrhage had led to an outpouring of adrenaline into the bloodstream, causing the severe constriction of her blood vessels, the extremely high blood pressure, and the racing of her heart. All these had been reversed by the phentolamine. This was a classic adrenaline storm, and I hoped we were now over the worst of it. As we lifted her off the X-ray table, Matthew raced in, waving the pink lab report.

"Eureka!" he shouted. "Hundreds of micrograms of adrenaline products per liter!"

Our surgeon, Aaron Weinberg, was waiting for us.

Alice smiled at him warmly. "Please be careful about the incision. I don't want an ugly scar on my tummy," she managed to whisper.

After completing his examination, Aaron took me aside. "The pheo is one thing, but her abdomen is tense and tender, particularly on the right. It's possible that her bowel has been damaged during the prolonged arterial constriction caused by the adrenaline. I'll have to extend the exploration of the abdominal cavity."

I understood what this might mean. "She is in your hands," I told him. "Do what needs to be done, but let's get her into surgery now."

Matthew and I, both half asleep by now, were in the operating theater two hours later as Aaron finished excising the large blood-tinged mass of the pheo.

"I don't like the look of the cecum," he said.

He was referring to the lower pouch-like end of the right side of the large bowel, the colon, from which the appendix arises. I peered over his shoulder and saw the angry, patchy purple discoloration of the intestinal wall.

"It's pregangrenous," he said. "This is what was hurting her. It was damaged by lack of blood flowing through its arteries before you got the phentolamine running. I'll have to take it out, do a right hemicolectomy. I hope she doesn't develop peritonitis. It's a pity we weren't able to operate sooner."

That was it. By noon she was in the recovery room, stable and sedated.

I went home for a few hours of sleep. Pam and Ben, who had been there throughout, now took over the vigil. A nurse was in attendance, but they refused to go home.

"Is it all over?" Pam asked me anxiously before I left. I saw that her eyes were red and swollen from a sleepless night of crying. She had taken her mother's sudden deterioration very badly. Despite her resentments, she was very attached to her mother and felt terribly guilty at not having heeded her complaints more seriously over the years.

"I shouldn't have listened to the doctors," Pam said. "I should have believed her. She knew what she was talking about. She always claimed it wasn't psychological and that they were all wrong, but I believed them and not her. And now if she should die, I will never forgive myself." Pam burst into tears.

I tried to assure her that none of this was her fault. "You must understand that you couldn't have done anything. After all, it was not that she avoided seeking medical help. She kept on going to doctors who just failed to make the correct diagnosis. There was nothing you could have done."

"You don't understand," she said. "I *am* guilty. My mother is the most selfish person who has ever lived. She was never there for me—not as a child, not as a teenager, not as an adult. Everything always centered on her. Other people see her as charming and interesting. I see her as a monster, a model of indifference to her family. Do you know that when I phoned to tell her that I had just been diagnosed with breast cancer and would have to have the surgery done within days, she was on her way to some party in Jerusalem? 'You must see that I can't let down the people who invited me,' she chirped. 'I'll come by on my way back from Jerusalem; we can talk then,' but then she never did. 'Sorry, dear, but we got back so late that there was no point' was all she had to say."

By this time Pam was sobbing so hard that even Ben was shaken out of his habitual calm and attempted to quiet her down. But she wouldn't stop talking. It came pouring out.

Finally, she must have felt that she had said too much. She clammed up and said quietly, "So you see, I am guilty. I resented her so much that I probably didn't care enough to question the doctors or believe her."

She left the room to wash her face and came back, more composed, a few minutes later. She then took over the watch for the next few hours.

I didn't want to tell Pam that I feared the next few days would be tricky. And so they were. Two days later Alice was running a fever and, despite massive antibiotics, developed an abscess under the right diaphragm. More surgery was clearly indicated. I wasn't sure how Alice would take the news, but she reacted with the same fortitude and cheerful resignation as before.

"If you think that after all this I'm going to let some microbe get the better of me, you don't know me," she said, looking in her hand mirror and smoothing down her hair. "I hope you can get all this done quickly, because I need to have my hair tinted before the end of the week if I'm to go to the party at the American ambassador's home next week. I'm not going to miss that dinner; it's going to be very stimulating."

I thought she must be joking. She was so sick; how could she possibly be thinking of a party when I was telling her she would have to have surgery again? Her white roots seemed to be bothering her more than the news I was conveying. But, no, she wasn't joking. She was perfectly serious. Could it be that such a bright woman could not understand the gravity of the situation? Thinking it over later, I came to the conclusion that her reaction was really in character. She had gone through life denying anything unpleasant and had contrived to pretend that it just didn't exist. Pam had always been exasperated by this characteristic. But at that moment, I thought Alice's amazing ability to think only positively was a blessing and might even be a decisive factor in her fight for recovery.

Unfortunately, she did not make it to the hairdresser or the party. The second operation to drain the abscess was done on day eight, and for a while everything seemed to be going well. Her fever subsided, and she showed signs of being on the way to recovery. My wife and I went out to dinner with some friends. On our way home, I suggested we pass by the hospital just to see how Alice was doing. I don't know what prompted this move; I just felt a kind of undefined anxiety. My wife was used to these bouts of intuition and encouraged me to go with my gut feeling. We arrived at the hospital at one o'clock in the morning.

I found her short of breath, and within minutes she was gasping for air. Our cardiologist's quick assessment showed a more ominous late sequel to the adrenaline storm she had weathered. Not only had her colon been damaged at the time, but her heart muscle too, as was now becoming evident. A loud murmur that had not been there before was now audible over her heart. One of her four heart valves was leaking badly with fluid building up in the lungs as a result, causing her severe shortness of breath; heart failure, in short. It looked like the pheo, our nemesis, was simply refusing to let her out of its grip. Although by now two weeks had gone by since its removal, its aftermath was still life-threatening.

Through the oxygen mask, en route to the cardiac intensive care unit, Alice whispered to me, "It seems that this odyssey refuses to end."

"Don't worry," I replied, "you'll beat this just as you beat everything else so far."

But this time I was far from sure. A small muscle within the heart cavity that normally assures proper closure of the valve had been severely damaged—stretched, in fact—during the storm.

"If the damaged muscle snaps, she will have to undergo surgery immediately," said Dr. Neufeld, our chief of cardiology.

So it looked as though Alice would have to undergo yet more and very hazardous surgery—this time an open-heart operation to replace the badly leaking mitral valve with an artificial prosthetic one, closing the leak.

"You understand how reluctant I am to make that recommendation right now, given her very precarious condition," said Neufeld. "It really is a touch-and-go situation, but I think we should give her a chance, using the right medications. Let's pray that if it doesn't tear, that little muscle will slowly heal and shrink back to its initial length. Hopefully this will minimize the leak. It's a chance we ought to take. Other cardiologists might not agree with this recommendation. It's a serious risk—but so is the alternative."

Alice spent the next three weeks in the intensive care unit, undergoing an intravenous infusion of drugs aimed at relieving the mechanical load on her failing heart. Amazingly, very slowly but steadily, the leak in the heart valve decreased in severity. In the fourth week, we were able to switch her to oral medication. By week six her shortness of breath was minimal and she was able to start moving around, walking several meters in her room. The valve leak had indeed nearly closed, the murmur barely audible now.

Throughout this ordeal she never once lost her faith in full recovery, actually encouraging those around her rather than looking to them for solace. At one stage she was hooked to a respirator and unable to talk. She indicated through a series of mimes that she wanted a Scrabble board and for the next three weeks communicated with everyone by moving letters on the board. The hospital staff was amazed by her courage, and I myself must admit that I have never had a patient who exhibited such fortitude in the face of such a catastrophic course of events.

Two and a half months after that mad car race to get her to the hospital, Pam and Ben were able to take Alice home. She had always been thin. Now a walking skeleton, she still insisted on having her hair done and face made up before allowing us to wheel her to the car. She improved steadily from then on. It took her three more months to rebuild enough muscle mass and strength to allow her a minimal amount of everyday activity. A year went by with a lot of medical follow-up and graded physical fitness rehabilitation, which she adhered to with grim determination. Finally, she was back to her former self—free of attacks and very proud of her achievement. In time she was able to stop all her heart medications and return to her old hectic lifestyle, which she still maintains today as a bright, energetic, and uncurbed eighty-five-year-old.

Her relationship with Pam has not changed despite the traumatic ordeal and Pam's guilt trip at the time. Alice's spoken and unspoken criticisms of her daughter are back, and Pam reacts with thinly veiled hostility, fueled by resentment and the long-rooted pain of a child who can never satisfy her mother. Alice feels vindicated, having proved that she was right and all her doctors wrong about her "neurosis." She has forbidden Pam and Ben to talk to anyone about the severity of her illness and passes it off as an unfortunate interlude in her life, which she has bracketed away as no longer relevant and "too boring."

I often think back to the decisions made by my fellow physicians who treated this woman. How could it have not occurred to any of the many doctors she saw in England over the years that she might indeed be harboring a pheochromocytoma? After all, the symptoms were classic, the appropriate diagnostic tests simple, noninvasive, and even inexpensive. Could it have been lack of knowledge? No way. British medical training was the best, always heavily oriented toward the importance of thorough and complete assessment of the clinical presentation of disease (signs and symptoms).

More likely there had been prejudgment of this patient's story toward the psychological or psychosomatic explanation because of her personality or the way she presented or conducted herself while talking to these practitioners. Indeed, I myself had experienced no small degree of exasperation in trying to get her to describe what she felt rather than what she thought or thought she knew. Could her demeanor have misled all those who had considered her case history?

It has been my own experience that not infrequently one encounters a patient with whom it is very difficult to establish rapport, to elicit a coherent story that one can follow appropriately in quest of a diagnosis. This is a failing of many physicians, which may lead to biased, prejudged opinions and generate flaws in the thoroughness and completeness of an evaluation. I cannot think of an alternative to this explanation for the failure of so many first-class physicians to suspect an obvious diagnostic possibility over such a prolonged period. The refusal of the London GP or my hospital colleague to consider the possibility of pheochromocytoma once explicitly presented to them seems to me to be of a totally different nature. Was it professional pride, first and foremost, a reluctance to acknowledge a colleague's suggestion as plausible merely because it had not occurred to them first? Or was it an emotionally triggered gap between an option that might be right and the choice of action they had decided upon? Or were they simply unwilling to consider that a rare reality they had never experienced until then was actually confronting them at that moment?

Whatever the psychological cause, a cognitive flaw shared by the medical community had nearly cost Alice her life. I shudder to think how often this phenomenon of prejudgment on the part of physicians takes place in everyday medical practice. Of course, a lot has changed in the way we physicians think and act since the 1970s. Modern technology, the litigiousness of our medical malpractice culture, and our heightened awareness of the politically correct have led to over- rather than underutilization of diagnostic procedures, and to more caution on the part of physicians to dismiss patients' stories that seem cranky or implausible. Still, I am not sure we have done enough to improve teaching of our students and trainees about the importance of questioning one's assumptions. Perhaps I am expecting the impossible. I am, however, sure that more introspection on the part of Alice's physicians would have considerably altered the course of this patient's life.

As for Alice herself, it is my belief that the hidden force that saw her through this severe, life-threatening ordeal was her deeply ingrained propensity to deny unpleasant realities. She had never for a moment considered the possibility of dying. From the first she was convinced that her illness was an unpleasant experience but not serious. Her spirits remained high even at the worst moments. I am convinced that this woman who exhibited such zest for making the most of life—often, it would seem, at the expense of her family—never relinquished her determination to continue living it to the hilt.

Alice fought her illness every step of the way, just as she today vigorously continues to fight old age, practically skipping along in her three-inch heels, her trim, youthful figure clothed in the latest fashion, meeting only young friends, keeping up with the latest innovations in bridge techniques, and even delighting in the use of a computer. She does not exhibit much interest in her grandchildren, or her great-grandchildren. They remind her too much of what she is attempting to forget—her eighty-five years of age.

9.

MY OWN MEDICINE

It happened as I was nearing the summit of the Schiesshorn, a mountain in the Swiss Alps that my wife, Ariela, and I climb every summer during our annual escape from the sultry July heat of Tel Aviv. This clear, brilliant morning I was alone, as Ariela had opted for a more relaxed day, with coffee and a good book rather than a one-thousand-meter, muscle-straining climbing ordeal.

Getting to the summit had become a tradition of sorts for us. Its highest point is marked by a two-meter-high wooden cross, held upright by a heavy mound of rocks that also holds a metal, watertight container the size of a shoebox. In summer, when the ice melts, the box lies visible to those reaching the summit. When we first opened it, we found the *gipfelbuch*, or summit register—a leather-bound notebook in which hikers have written a few lines in numerous languages, recording the thoughts and feelings sparked by the magnificent full-circle panorama below. Our own contributions over the years had been to record the birth of each one of our ten grandchildren, adding a prayer for their well-being. These were the only entries in Hebrew throughout the entire register, begun in the late 1970s.

As I gazed down across the valley at the spectacular view, I suddenly noticed my vision was blurred. After blinking away some tears brought on by traces of sunscreen mixed with drops of sweat, I took a more careful look at the outlines of the mountain peaks on the other side of the valley and saw two mountains where moments ago there had only been one. I realized immediately that I was experiencing double vision, or diplopia.

This was new to me, and disconcerting, to say the least. I'd long known my eyes weren't perfect. I'd had glaucoma for many years, the result of bad genes inherited from both my parents, topped by a squash-ball injury to my right eye sustained during my fellowship at UCSF in the 1970s. But the pressure in both eyes had always been well controlled by a variety of eye drops, and there had been no deleterious effect on my vision to date.

Although not an ophthalmologist, I knew very well as a general internist that the sudden occurrence of double vision had nothing to do with glaucoma. Its grimmer implications, I thought at that moment, could be neurological. This was scary. Could something be going wrong in my brain—here, now, with nobody around to help me? Sitting down on a rock, I forced myself to take a deep breath and calm down. After a few minutes, I felt more composed and proceeded to do as careful an assessment of the situation as I could manage.

I quickly determined that other than the double vision, nothing was manifestly wrong with my head. There was no dizziness, headache, or other sensory symptom. I was moving all four limbs freely. My muscle strength—which I tested with a few easy push-ups and rising from squatting to a standing position—was intact. So was my sense of balance and equilibrium, which I checked by standing first on one foot then on the other, with both eyes shut.

More at ease though still bewildered, I shifted my attention to the diplopia itself. I quickly determined that it disappeared if I kept my right eye shut. I verified this by repeatedly observing the view with one eye closed, alternating between the right eye and the left.

I sat down again to ponder what all this meant. It seemed to me it was somehow related to the small muscles of the eyeball. I soon built a worst-case scenario wherein being sixty-five years old, I was possibly experiencing a brain TIA (transient ischemic attack), otherwise known as a minimal near-stroke. Such strokes result from a sudden temporary blockage of the blood supply to a particular area of the brain, usually due to the passage through an artery of a small blood clot or cholesterol crumb. TIA symptoms may last for minutes or several hours at most and then recede with no evident residual damage. That is why they are termed "transient." However, they may portend a real stroke, with its ensuing long-term, often permanent consequences.

Yet I knew that the symptom—double vision related to one eye—was not typical of TIA. I had none of the usual symptoms—no weakness in a limb or transient blindness or blind spots in one eye. Besides, I was in excellent health, fit and lean, and doing daily aerobic exercise. I had quit a mild smoking habit more than thirty years earlier and bore no risk factors for heart or blood vessel disease. My blood pressure, cholesterol, and sugar levels were all normal, and even my genes were OK in this respect. "No," I concluded, mulling all this over, "I don't know what it is, but it's most likely not a TIA."

What then should I do about it? A few more moments of thought yielded what I considered to be the most practical decision—that is, to plan and execute my own treatment, at least for the time being. Obviously, I'd have to be examined properly, but any visits to the doctor and subsequent diagnostics could wait until after our vacation. For the moment, on the off chance that it was a TIA after all, I would start taking a daily tablet of aspirin, the accepted treatment used to prevent further episodes.

Rather pleased with myself for having devised this conservative course of action, I proceeded to hike down the mountain. I made it down without mishap, keeping my right eye shut for most of the two-hour descent. By the time I reached the village, some three hours after the event on the mountaintop, the double vision had disappeared. After a stop at the local pharmacy for aspirin tablets, I walked slowly back to our hotel.

Ariela was waiting for me anxiously. "Where have you been?" she said. "What kept you so long? You had me so worried. I was about to set out to look for you."

Ariela is a worrier. As she herself puts it, she tends to overprotect me from myself. I knew full well that if I told her the story, she'd have us return home posthaste, cutting short a holiday we'd both looked forward to for a whole year. Seeing her response, I was even happier with my decision not to tell her anything.

"There was no need to worry," I assured her. "I didn't encounter any prowling bears, and there was no avalanche. My climb just took a little longer than usual. I probably just stopped more often to enjoy the stupendous views several times along the way and didn't notice the time. Sorry."

Ariela has a sharp nose for possible deception. She fixed me with a suspicious glare. "Are you sure you're telling me everything?"

"Of course I am," I said breezily. "Let's go down to the lake and have some tea and raspberry tart."

My wife is mad about these delicately baked crusts, filled with fresh raspberries and topped with a dab of whipped cream; they'd be just the thing to distract her. We walked down to the lakeside café and sat at a table under a tree to watch the late-afternoon light on the water.

Children floated little boats, and a lone swan glided elegantly by, followed at some distance by a mother duck and her retinue of ducklings. All was supremely peaceful. The double vision was gone, and I was feeling fine. Perhaps, I thought to myself, I had imagined the whole thing.

Over the next few days, I observed myself carefully, with some trepidation that I thought I was hiding successfully. One day, however, as I surreptitiously checked my vision by closing an eye, Ariela suddenly demanded, "Why are you squinting like that?"

"I wasn't squinting; something got into my eye," I replied, making a mental note to be more careful when she was around.

"Are you sure? I've noticed you doing that several times in the last few days."

"Nonsense," I said in my most irritated voice, intent on stopping the questioning. "I'm fine."

And I truly was. I kept taking the aspirin every morning as planned, and the rest of the holiday passed without incident.

Back home again, in keeping with my original decision, I embarked on a very thorough series of specialist consultations and tests. This was easy for me to organize with my colleagues at the hospital without breaking my routine schedule or tipping off my wife. I was seen by ophthalmologists, neurologists, blood vessel specialists, and cardiologists; none of them found any evidence of potential causes or signs of a recent TIA. Possibly a fleeting blood-vessel spasm was the neuro-ophthalmologist's suggestion.

Both she and the neurologist strongly recommended a brain MRI scan to look for signs of any blood-vessel related event, either recent or more remote (and unfelt) that might shed light on what had happened on the mountain. I declined the proposal, knowing that an MRI might well cause more uncertainty and often has no practical significance in regard to treatment. After all, in perfectly healthy people my age, MRIs often reveal brain lesions that have no explanation. In any case, I was already undergoing the preventive treatment that follows positive MRIs, taking aspirin in such low doses that its benefits far outweighed any possible adverse effects. My neurologist grudgingly went along with my analysis and conclusions, and I happily put the episode behind me and got back to my daily routine.

At home, however, Ariela still sensed I was hiding a health problem from her.

"What are you denying now?" she demanded.

"Nothing. I'm not a denier."

"Sure you are. Your specialty is making molehills out of mountains. I remember the time you had typhoid fever and kept insisting it was just a passing virus. 'Nothing to get worried about,' you said. You strictly forbade me to call in a doctor, claiming you could treat yourself. Finally, when you got worse, I decided to override your wishes and called Eitan, who berated me for not having called him earlier. He felt your swollen spleen, diagnosed typhoid, and took you to the hospital. Remember that?" she said triumphantly. "I decided then and there never again to go along with your 'rational' diagnoses when it concerns your own health, and in the future to act according to my own common sense."

"That was different," I protested weakly.

"Oh yes? And what about the time you passed out in the theater in London when you had one of your fainting spells? Remember how you forgot to tell me until I happened to find out about it a year later?"

That was indeed a strange incident. We had gone to see *King Lear* at the Barbican together with Ariela's cousin. That evening I had a low-grade virus, but loath to miss the great performance of the Royal Shakespeare Company, I took a couple of aspirins and we went to the show. I began feeling a little queasy after the gory, very realistic portrayal onstage of Gloucester's eyes being poked out. The intermission took place right after that scene. Ariela and her cousin led the way to the bar. Following behind, I was separated from them in the crowded aisle. Then I suddenly passed out. When I opened my eyes a few seconds later, I found myself lying flat on my back, with a crowd of concerned people bending over me. The theater usher wanted to call an ambulance, but I wasn't alarmed. I've always had this tendency to pass out in reaction to even minor situations of physical stress, such as spraining an ankle or contracting a nasty stomach virus.

"No way," I told the usher. "I'm a physician. This happens to me quite often. There's really no need for any further ado."

After signing a waiver, I went to the men's room, washed my face, and then joined Ariela and her cousin in the bar. They had not noticed anything, and I saw no reason to upset them by relating the whole incident. We sat through the performance and got back safely to the hotel. The next day I was fine, and later on forgot all about that trivial incident. It was more than a year before I made the mistake of telling my wife about it.

Now, however, I saw I could not win this one. Rather than have Ariela dredge up all her stories of my past withholdings, I gave way and told her what had happened on the mountain.

She was furious. "I will never believe you again," she said, storming off. When she calmed down, she made me promise never to hide anything from her again. I made the promise, naturally, for the sake of peace and quiet, but had little intention of keeping it.

An uneventful year went by, including the traditional two-week stint in the Alps hiking the mountain trails as we have always done. Then, back at home, while taking a stroll with Ariela in the late afternoon of Yom Kippur, the Day of Atonement, I suddenly lost vision in my right eye. Its entire field of vision was riddled with black holes. This time too there were no other symptoms whatsoever. Ariela immediately put me in the car and drove me to the hospital. It was eerie; as always on Yom Kippur, the country had come to a standstill, and not a single other car besides ours was to be seen on the empty roads.

Twenty minutes after the episode began, we arrived at the ophthalmology ER. It too was empty, devoid of the usual bustle of harassed doctors, nurses, and worried patients. There was only one tired and hungry resident, who had been fasting since the previous evening and on duty all night. He examined my eyes carefully and could see nothing out of the ordinary. In fact, by the time he completed his examination, my vision was back to normal.

The next day the neuro-ophthalmologist, whose examination again yielded no findings, repeated her suggestion of an MRI of the brain. Once again I politely declined, for the same reasons as before. Once again I was put through the diagnostic process, and again it turned out entirely negative—almost. This time the cardiologist noticed on the echocardiogram a minimal mitral valve prolapse (MVP), a slight abnormality of one of my heart valves. In fact, it was so slight as to be considered only a variant of the normal anatomy. Nevertheless, given my recent history and the propensity of MVP to send the occasional tiny clot into the arteries leading to the brain, the cardiologist felt that continuing the daily aspirin would be prudent. The neuro-ophthalmologist concurred, and I went on with the regimen. The following days and weeks were fine, and life continued apace.

Two more years went by. I was very busy supervising a major research program we were initiating at the hospital, and heavily involved in putting together a new course I was to teach at our graduate school on the science of new drug development (my specialty being clinical pharmacology, the science of the rational use of drugs, what they do to our body, and what our body does to them). At some point I noticed I was having some daily headaches, which, though mild, were bad enough to make me take the occasional Tylenol. Never having been a headachy person, I was surprised, but not unduly worried.

Several days later at work, the headache was worse. Thinking that workload-related high blood pressure could well be the cause, I asked a colleague to check it. The reading was normal. As the headaches could be suppressed on one or two Tylenol a day, I stopped thinking about them and went on with my work. Despite my promise, I did not mention any of this to Ariela. No point in worrying her needlessly, I told myself. Nor could I identify a possible connection between these headaches and my previous eye problems, and I therefore did not consult with any of my doctors who had been so thorough in trying to makes sense of them at the time.

Two weeks after the onset of the headaches, there were new developments. I noticed recurrent bouts of tingling sensations running down my right arm from shoulder to fingertips, lasting seconds at first, and eventually a minute or so. As these often occurred when I was working at the computer, I shrugged them off as being related to my poor posture at the keyboard. I tried to relieve them by flexing my fingers, clenching my fists, and moving my arm about at the shoulder and elbow.

Many months later a colleague told me of a conversation he'd had with me at the time. He had noticed something was bothering me. When he asked if anything was wrong, I jokingly replied I hoped I wasn't getting a stroke, but didn't elaborate. Interestingly, I had no recollection either of the conversation or of having had such thoughts.

The tingles continued, but the headaches had somehow subsided. Again, I succeeded in relegating the story to deep storage, giving the symptoms no further thought. I was very excited by the work on the new course, which was a first at our medical school and involved bringing in academics from two other schools in Israel, as well as people from the pharmaceutical industry in Israel and abroad. I had invested a lot of work and enthusiasm in the project but was also feeling anxious, uncertain that its goals would be achieved. The success of the course was my overriding concern, and it drove out all smaller, more negligible issues, such as tingling sensations in my arm.

Things came to a head on a Saturday, a few days after my conversation with my concerned friend. As usual, Ariela and I walked to the cemetery on the weekend to look after her father's grave. When we got back home, standing at the doorway, I took out my keys but found myself unable to insert the key into the lock. There was also a sensation of weakness in my leg, and all of a sudden I felt disoriented.

"I think I'm having a stroke," I said. "Get me some aspirin."

Ariela brought me the pills, and I downed a full dose while she got out the car. We live quite near the hospital, and the ride took only six or seven minutes.

This was a first for me, being wheeled into the emergency ward as a patient. They all knew me—the reception clerks, nurses, and most of the doctors on duty, many of whom had been my students or trainees. It was strange to be questioned, probed, and looked at by those whom I had taught over so many years. On the other hand, their serious but warm and caring demeanor gave me a much-needed sense of confidence. Something was seriously wrong, obviously, but I was in good hands.

The neurology resident completed his history taking, carefully recording the story of my past transient vision problems. The physical exam confirmed a slight weakness of the muscles of my right thigh and leg. He sent me at once to radiology for computed tomography (CT) of the head.

As I was rolled out of the machine's tunnel, Ariela and I were courteously invited to view the pictures with the grave-faced radiologist and neurologist. As I sat there in my wheelchair, the four of us stared unbelievingly at the screened images. A very big mass inside my skull, similar in size and shape to a squashed tennis ball, capped and compressed the surface of the left hemisphere of my brain, pushing it well over the midline, toward the right. This subdural hematoma, as it is called, was a massive collection of partially clotted blood that had congealed and expanded in the space within the skull, between its thick inner lining, the dura, and the surface of the brain itself. It looked as though it had been there for some time—several months or more, the neurologist thought—slowly building up to its current size.

"Have you suffered any headaches lately?" he asked.

"No," I answered, completely forgetting the headaches that had troubled me in the preceding weeks. Since I had not told Ariela about them, she could not correct this omission, and the medical record failed to mention the presence of headaches in the weeks preceding the event.

"Could you try to recollect any head trauma, even minor, you may have sustained over the last year?" he persisted.

I knew what he was thinking. Often these chronic hematomas result from minimal blows to the head. While the patient may not even recall them, they nevertheless cause a slow but continuous oozing of blood from injured small blood vessels into the skull cavity.

"No, I can't remember any such incident," I said.

"Do you have a history of a bleeding tendency?"

"None."

"Well, then," he concluded, "it's probably the aspirin you've been taking."

I was stunned. I had not expected—or rather, had led myself not to expect—any serious findings this time either, let alone this suggested explanation of what we were looking at. With the past episodes related to my eye, I had been dreading the possibility of a stroke or some such event. And like all the specialists who'd seen me, I knew that given even the remote possibility of my having sustained a TIA in the past, I ought to take aspirin for its beneficial effects in preventing a subsequent stroke. Hence the small daily dose for two years.

The additional single large dose that I took this time before leaving home for the hospital was the prescribed self-medication recommended for strokes or similar emergencies. But my own case, as it turned out, was not one of those. Not only was aspirin not helpful, but I was hit by its worst adverse effect: its propensity to cause major bleeding episodes, including the rare phenomenon (described in only one in roughly ten thousand patients) of bleeding into the skull cavity, or, even worse, into the brain tissue itself.

In truth, I should have suspected something of the sort much earlier. All the signs of a process of a mass developing in my skull had been there all along. Had it been a patient presenting the same sequence of symptoms, I would doubtlessly have sent him or her to have a CT scan and had the diagnosis confirmed almost immediately. The subdural hematoma clearly explained all the symptoms I'd been dismissing so casually: first the headaches and then the episodes of tingling—clearly a form of seizure manifesting not as convulsions but as bouts of aberrant sensations. Ultimately, the mounting pressure on my brain had caused the disorientation and weakness in my leg that finally brought me to the hospital. As it turned out, taking that extra dose of aspirin was the worst thing I could have done, since it sent a fresh, large surge of blood into the area already occupied by the hematoma.

Meanwhile, my eldest son, Amir, a cardiologist himself, had joined Ariela at my bedside in the ER cubicle. Thanks to their presence, and my trust in the nurses and doctors looking after me, a sort of peace of mind settled over me, and an assurance that all would be well. I was put on an IV drip and loaded up with antiepileptic medication to abort any worsening of the seizure disorder. The neurologist then called in the neurosurgeons and they took over. It was clear that I was going to need surgery, burr holes drilled into my skull to allow the hematoma to be suctioned out. They thought it wise, however, to wait a few days in order to allow the effect of the full dose of aspirin I had so unwisely taken to wear off at least partially, as it could cause further bleeding during or after the operation.

In preparation for the surgery, I was put through the usual procedure of admission to the neurosurgery ward. First, a young doctor again took down my medical history, which was pretty dull since I had never had any ailment that I could remember. He too asked me about recent headaches, and again I could not recall having had any.

I spent the night in the hospital, and by the next morning was feeling much better. The tingling sensations were gone, and the weakness in my leg barely noticeable. I was a bit groggy from the antiepileptic medication I was now taking orally, but other than that felt reasonably well. In view of my stable condition, the surgeons decided they could stick with the original plan and scheduled the operation for three days later. Moreover, as there had been an outbreak of cases of postoperative wound infections on the ward, they allowed me to go home for the nights and return daily to be checked during the morning rounds.

The next day at home was uneventful. The anticonvulsive pills were still preventing the tingling, and the only discomfort was in the waiting.

But the following morning, as she helped me walk to the toilet, Ariela noticed that my gait was unsteady.

"What's wrong?" she asked. "You're walking with your feet spread apart, as if trying to keep yourself from falling."

"That's just a side effect of the antiepileptic pills—probably an overdose following the huge infusion they gave me in the ER the day before yesterday," I reassured her.

"Oh no, you don't," she said. "We are going to the hospital right now."

I was too weak to argue, and off we went. At the hospital the surgeons fully concurred with Ariela. After a blood test showed normal drug levels, ruling out my overdose theory, they decided that the burr-holes operation should not be delayed any longer.

The anesthetist came to see me, and she too took my medical history. "Didn't you have any headaches while all this was building up?" she asked.

"None," I answered quite sincerely. I had simply erased them from my memory.

The operation went well, although the surgeon reported that he'd had unusual difficulty in drilling through my skull bones, as if they were thicker than their usual double plating, overlying the large hematoma. In fact, he found that the outer layer of the hematoma mass had become partially calcified, acquiring bone-like consistency—yet another sign of just how long it had been sitting there, silently growing. The surgeon told us he'd been able to remove the most bothersome bone-like fragments left in the cavity after the drilling. However, he added, some remained. These, it turned out, were to prove quite problematic.

As expected, by the next day all my symptoms were gone. I was walking normally, and even the grogginess had disappeared. Feeling so much better, I was truly relieved when one day later I was allowed to go home for the weekend. As it turned out, however, my troubles were far from over. After a restful first night in my own bed, I was enjoying the company of a friend and colleague of many years who'd come from Jerusalem to visit me. We were talking about my physician-to-patient transfiguration, its strangeness and the inherent feeling of helplessness, of having relinquished control of my own fate after a lifetime of being responsible for that of others. Suddenly, in midsentence, I lost my ability to speak. I knew what I was trying to say but could only utter incoherent monosyllabic sounds. Deeply alarmed, my friend and Ariela quickly piled me into the car and we headed back to the hospital.

There are two versions of my reaction to this new emergency. I recall myself as concerned but calm and controlled, with no sense of panic or fear. According to Ariela and my friend, however, I was extremely distressed throughout the drive, and kept pounding my fist into my hand in frustration at my helplessness as I repeatedly tried, and repeatedly failed, to convey something to them.

Back at the hospital, I was taken immediately to the CT suite. The scan now revealed massive fresh bleeding into the cavity left after the burr-hole drainage of the original hematoma. With no further ado, I was rushed to the operating theater. After priming with a transfusion of blood platelets (guaranteed free of aspirin effects), I was wheeled in for more surgery. This time it was a full craniotomy, which involved raising a large semicircular flap of the scalp and bones overlying the location of the old hematoma and exposing the brain surface through the large opening in the skull. The surgeon was thus able to clean out the new, big blood clot and meticulously remove the last few small fragments left behind at the first operation. He was also now able to cauterize the small blood vessels and stop the oozing that was the cause of this latest complication.

This time round he was very satisfied with the results. "It's that thick skull of his," he told my wife jokingly. "We all know him to be one of our more hardheaded people when it comes to medical issues, but I would never have thought I'd run into his obstinate skull bones using my surgical instruments, let alone have them complicate a simple burr-hole procedure!"

Jokes aside, he believed that the bony fragments left behind the first time may have caused the additional blood vessel injury and renewed bleeding that mandated the second, bigger operation.

I spent the next forty-eight hours in intensive care. While I know Ariela was at my bedside most of the time, little else remained imprinted in my mind. Indeed, in the ensuing weeks I often complained how surprising it was that this or that friend or coworker hadn't taken the trouble to stop by and offer their good wishes. My grumblings caused Ariela much mirth; each and every person I was so angry with, she told me, had in fact come to see me at the ICU, most of them more than once. Retrograde amnesia, they call it. My mind was erasing or burying the memories of what had happened, or, perhaps, of what *might* have happened had circumstances not forced me to deal with what was going on in my head.

The one scene I remember clearly is waking up at some hour of darkness (night and day are often confused by the on/off rhythms of lighting in the ICU) with IV lines dripping fluids into my arm and a rubber catheter draining my urinary bladder and causing me the greatest discomfort I'd had since it all began—even greater than that caused by the knocks my skull bones had taken. Looking around I realized someone was there at the bedside, sitting quietly in the dark. It was my son Mike, the more emotional among my three, but, like his brothers, not given to much demonstrativeness.

"What time is it?" I asked. "What are you doing here, Mike?"

"It's three a.m.," he said quietly. "I couldn't sleep, so I drove to the hospital and have been sitting here with you."

Probably sensing the rush of my emotion, my feeling of security and warmth generated by his being there, he said no more and just took my hand in his. I slipped back into a deep, peaceful sleep.

Back on the ward, my recovery over the next few days was rapid and complete, with all the symptoms gone, hopefully for good. I was allowed to leave the hospital and recuperate at home. The healing process took its time. Now and then I still found myself unable to speak, and still felt recurrent tingling in my arm and fingers. These were to be expected, as the aftereffects of the pressure on the brain tissue, which had been there for months, would take quite a few weeks to recede.

For this very reason, it was made clear to me I would have to continue taking full doses of antiepileptic medication for at least six months and possibly up to a year. These drugs took a lot of getting used to and had several unpleasant side effects, such as loss of concentration and a slight tremor that appeared in my right hand. I pored over the medical literature concerning the management of this type of epilepsy and haggled vigorously with the neurologists over the required duration and dosage. Finally, I prevailed: the sentence was mitigated to three months and the doses lowered. Consequently, I was able to return to part-time work four weeks after the operation, and when the treatment period was complete, I was already back at the office full-time.

It was now time to answer the question of the aspirin. Did the bleeding episode rule out any future use of aspirin or aspirin-like drug, should the need arise? Or should the taking of aspirin be renewed now, given the remote possibility of past TIAs?

The latter question was easy to answer.

"Let's do the MRI of the brain now," said the neurologist. "The one you were dead against when you had those vision problems, remember? If it shows no TIA lesions in the brain tissue itself, we'll know for sure that you never needed the aspirin in the first place and certainly don't need it now."

His words hit me like a bolt from the blue. How right he was now—and how wrong I'd been then! I had turned down the MRI for fear of discovering lesions that wouldn't help establish a diagnosis and wouldn't make decisions any easier. But I had neglected to even consider the possibility that a completely negative scan showing no TIA lesions would have completely ruled out a past TIA event. Had I known the facts, I would never have started taking the aspirin! And I thought I was being so clever; what a price to pay for such hubris.

The MRI showed no lesions at all in the brain tissue, only the residue of the subdural hematoma and the surgeries. "How typical of a clinical pharmacologist—self-medicating for the wrong reason and suffering one of the drug's rarest adverse effects," the neurologist teased me. "And by the way, we still don't know what caused that double vision on the mountain."

All I could do was shrug and smile rather sheepishly.

Today the only external reminder of the entire ordeal is my new cropped hairstyle, designed to conceal the furrowed scar crossing my skull. This has had the added bonus of being very much in fashion, judging by the similar haircuts sported by my sons and the appreciative input from my daughter and her friends.

The internal reminders of what I went through will probably always be there. First, there is a newfound humility. After a lifetime of treating and advising others in often dire circumstances, here I was, on the receiving end, in a similarly precarious state. There is also a new acute awareness of my own vulnerability. For years I had prided myself on my fitness and excellent health, which I sincerely thought would last forever, only to be rudely introduced to the frailties of my own body.

But above all, there is the acknowledgement of my own failure as a physician. I, who have guided so many patients through extremely tough decisions, had made a series of foolhardy decisions myself. Not only had I decided to self-medicate—something I would never have recommended to a fellow doctor—but I subsequently refused to follow the advice of my colleagues. I had declined the MRI years earlier, on my own subjective judgment. The scan would have put to rest the TIA hypothesis. I would never have taken the aspirin, and the rest would not have been history.

Ariela claims that my behavior throughout was a form of denial, stemming from the fact that I couldn't face the possibility of an imminent stroke. Only a denier, she contends, would have disregarded for so long the warning signals—the headaches, the tingling arms. Only a denier would have completely wiped some of them from his mind. And who else would insist, as I still do, that the initial event was never really dangerous, that the loss of the power of speech was "transitory," or that the craniotomy was not life-threatening or even worrisome?

While it's unlikely I'll ever give Ariela the pleasure of confessing I'm a denier, I will never again resort to self-diagnosis or self-medication. "Physician, heal thyself" should not be taken literally. I certainly learned this the hard way.

Made in the USA
Charleston, SC
03 December 2013